Your New Baby

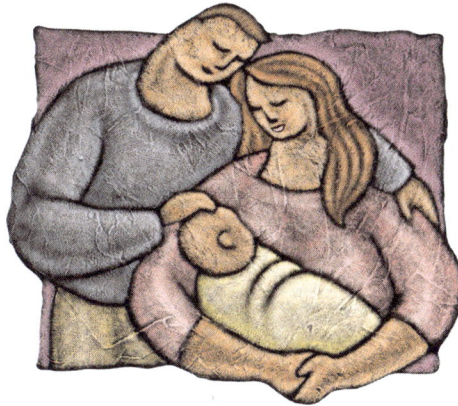

Angela Nicoletti, RNC, WHNP

Author of Educational Materials
Pediatric and Adolescent Gynecology

Publisher
The Goodheart-Willcox Company, Inc.
Tinley Park, Illinois

2

Library of Congress Catalog Card Number 2008051974

ISBN 978-1-60525-127-1

1 2 3 4 5 6 7 8 9 – 10 – 14 13 12 11 10 09

Library of Congress Cataloging-in-Publication Data

Nicoletti, Angela.
    Your new baby / Angela Nicoletti.
        p. cm.
    Includes index.
    ISBN 978-1-60525-127-1
    1. Teenage pregnancy. 2. Teenage mothers. 3. Parenting. I. Title.
RG556.5.N535 2010
649'.122--dc22
                                                                    2008051974

About the Author

Angela Nicoletti is an author of educational materials, a consultant to video producers and textbook developers, and a Section Editor for the Journal of Pediatric and Adolescent Gynecology.

Formerly, Angela served as Clinical Coordinator of the Adolescent Reproductive Health Services (ARHS) at Brigham and Women's Hospital in Boston, Massachusetts, a provider of health care to pregnant and parenting teens. She also served as a lecturer in the Graduate School of Nursing of Boston College. Angela, who holds a master's degree in nursing, has presented numerous papers on teen pregnancy, breast-feeding, maternal attachment, and teen development.

Angela's professional contributions also include her service to: the Adolescent Health Committee of the American College of Obstetrics and Gynecology; the Practice Committee of the Association of Women's Health, Obstetrics, and Neonatal Nursing; the board of directors for the National Organization of Adolescent Pregnancy Parenting and Prevention; and the Massachusetts Alliance for Young Families.

4

Acknowledgments

We would like to thank the following professionals who reviewed the original text and provided valuable input:

Cathy Allison
GRADS Coordinator
Auburn Career Center
Concord, Ohio

Dawn Gale Aspacher
Parent Educator
Child and Family Resources, Inc.
  The Center for Adolescent
  Parents
Tucson, Arizona

JoAnn J. Bartek
FCS Teacher/Director,
  Student Parent Team SCLC
Lincoln High School
Lincoln, Nebraska

Martha Hamdani-Swain
former Program Coordinator,
Pregnancy Education and
  Parenting Program
Jack Yates High School
Houston, Texas

Sheree M. Moser
FCS Department Chair and
  District Assistant
Lincoln High School
Lincoln, Nebraska

Sara McDonald Rohar
Project Director,
  Young Mother's Program
Birmingham City Schools
Birmingham, Alabama

Table of Contents

Chapter 5
Exercising and Eating Right 85

Chapter 6
Preparing for the New Arrival 101

Chapter 7
Experiencing Childbirth 122

Chapter 8
New Mom, New Baby 139

Introduction

Few times in life will you be faced with more change than when you find out you or your partner are pregnant. Pregnancy means a major adjustment for you. As a young person, you may not have planned to make all these transitions so soon, yet here you are. Perhaps you didn't want to be involved in a pregnancy right now. If you are, though, make the most of this experience and enjoy it as much as you can. Learning about the changes that lie ahead can help you do just that.

Your New Baby was written with you in mind. The goal of this book is to take some of the fear and mystery out of pregnancy and childbirth by explaining these subjects in language that is easy to understand. It covers many topics, including the following:

- prenatal health care and lifestyle habits during pregnancy
- preparations for parenthood or adoption
- labor and delivery
- newborn care

The language in this book is directed to pregnant teens because it is the young women who experience the physical changes of pregnancy, labor, and delivery. However, fathers-to-be can gain much by reading this book, too. They will learn how to be supportive of the mother-to-be and how to care for a newborn. A father's support and involvement are very important to his partner, his baby, and himself.

Your baby may be a girl or a boy. To make the chapters easier to read, we have referred to your baby in some sections as he and in other sections as she. We hope this will also help you relate to the chapters in a personal way as you think about your baby. We encourage you to do all you can to have a healthy pregnancy and a healthy baby!

Chapter 1
How It All Begins

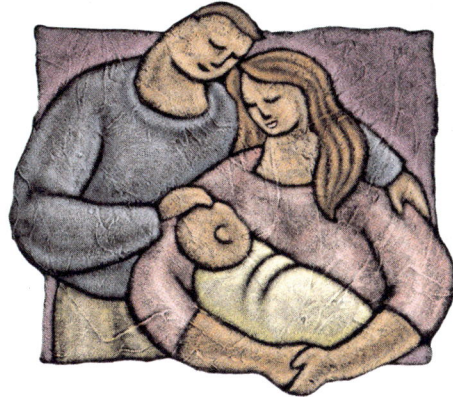

It seems so simple—a woman becomes pregnant, and nine months later a baby is born. Of course, it is a much more complex process than that! You may have questions about how pregnancy occurs. To understand this process, you must first learn how the male and female reproductive systems work.

The Reproductive Systems

The reproductive system includes the parts and pathways that allow a person to bear children. This system forms even before birth. For the first few years, the reproductive system is not very active. Changes begin during the late childhood or early teen years. These changes are part of a process called puberty. Through this process, a person's reproductive organs mature and become able to create new life.

The reproductive systems of a man and a woman differ. Both are needed to create a new human being. For this reason, you should learn how both systems work. This will give you a better picture of how pregnancy begins.

The Male Reproductive System

The male reproductive system has many parts. See Figure 1-1. Most are internal (inside the body). Others are external (outside the body). Each part plays a role in a man's ability to father a child.

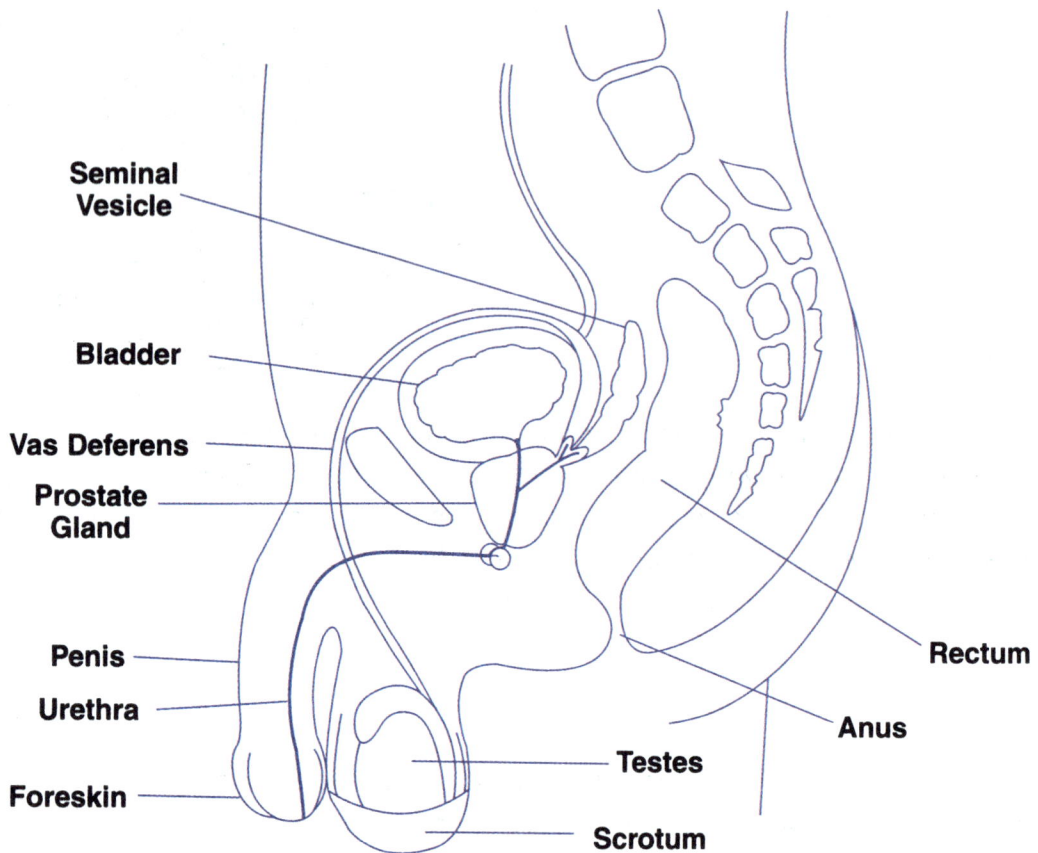

1-1 This side view shows all the major organs of the male reproductive system.

These parts work together to create, store, and transport the male reproductive cell. This cell is called a sperm. This cell's function is to unite with the woman's egg cell inside her body to create a baby.

Sperm are very tiny—they measure only $1/500$ of an inch. They are so small they cannot be seen without a microscope. Each sperm has the following three parts:

☛ a head that penetrates egg cells. The head contains genetic material to be passed from the man to his children. See Figure 1-2.

☛ a midsection that stores energy the sperm will need to swim toward the egg cell inside the woman's body.

☛ a whiplike tail that helps the sperm swim very quickly.

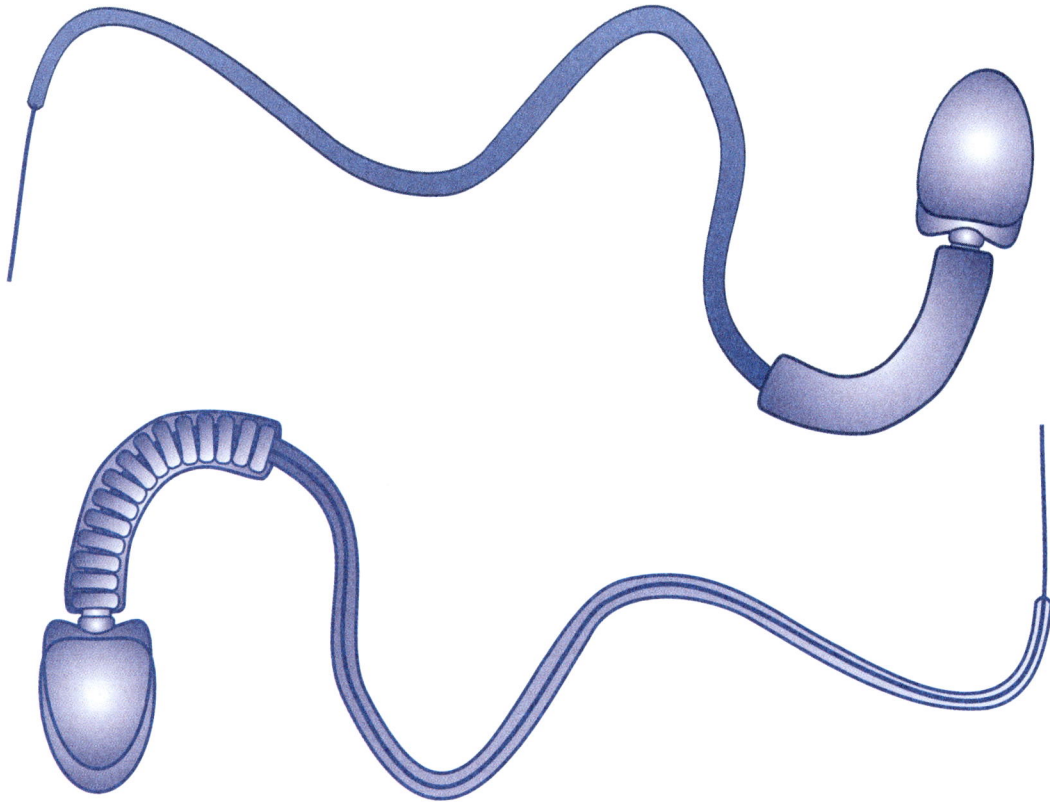

1-2 Can you identify the three parts of the sperm cell from this drawing?

A man's body starts making sperm at puberty. At this time, the hormone testosterone signals his body to begin making sperm. Testosterone also controls body changes in males. These include hair growth, voice deepening, and muscle development. Once sperm development begins, it will continue until old age.

Both testosterone and sperm are produced by the testes. The testes are two small, walnut-shaped organs. They are located inside the scrotum. The scrotum is a sac of loose skin that hangs down just behind the penis. The scrotum protects the testes. It keeps them at the right temperature. To produce sperm, the testes must be a few degrees cooler than the rest of the body. The scrotum can contract to move the testes close to the body for warmth. It can relax to move the testes away from the body for cooling.

After sperm are produced, they must mature (finish developing). Sperm leave the testes and begin their path through the male reproductive system. Their next stop is the epididymis (eh-pih-DIH-dih-mihs). This is a very long tube that is curled up inside a firm sack. Here the sperm reach maturity. Once they are mature, sperm travel into two long, thin tubes called the vas deferens (vas DEHF-uh-ruhnz). Here they are stored until they are released from the body. Each vas deferens can hold several million sperm.

When sperm are to be released from the body, they leave the vas deferens and travel through the rest of the reproductive system. Two glands called the seminal vesicles (SEHM-ih-nuhl VEH-sihk-uhls) add fluid to the sperm. Another fluid is added to the sperm by the prostate gland. This is a plum-sized gland that sits just beneath the bladder. This mixture of sperm and fluid is called semen. The semen is then sent into the ejaculatory duct. The ejaculatory duct is a small duct that connects the seminal vesicles to the urethra. The urethra (yoo-REE-thruh) is the tube inside the penis that carries urine from the bladder out of the body. It also carries semen from the ejaculatory duct to the outside of the body. Urine and semen cannot be in the urethra at the same time. During sexual activity, the prostate gland blocks the urethra, keeping urine out.

The urethra carries semen outside the body through a process called ejaculation. Semen is released from the body when a male ejaculates. A series of muscle contractions push the semen out of the penis through the urethra. The purpose of ejaculation is to deliver sperm (contained in the semen) to the woman's body. Inside her body, the sperm swim quickly to find an egg to fertilize. Sperm can live inside the woman's body for as long as three days.

The penis is the most obvious part of the male reproductive system. Semen and urine exit the male's body through the penis (but not at the same time). The penis is the part of a man's body that enters the woman's body during sexual intercourse.

The penis has three parts—the shaft, glans, and foreskin. The shaft is the long part. Inside the shaft are the urethra and three cylinders of a special spongy tissue. When a male is sexually aroused, this tissue fills with blood. This causes the penis to become harder, wider, and longer. This is called an erection. When a man is not sexually aroused, the penis is softer, shorter, and smaller.

The glans is the smooth, round tip of the penis. It has many nerve endings. The glans is very sensitive to touch. The opening of the urethra is inside the tip of the glans.

The foreskin is the looser skin that covers the penis. Sometimes part of the foreskin is removed. This is done in an operation called circumcision. (Circumcision is described in more detail in Chapter 8.)

Now you have learned the major parts of the male reproductive system. Return to Figure 1-1. Trace the path of the sperm again, naming each part of the system. The male reproductive system is only half of the story, however. The female reproductive system is just as essential in creating new life.

The Female Reproductive System

The female reproductive system allows a woman to have children. It is a group of many parts that work together. Some parts are external and others are internal. See Figure 1-3. This system has three main purposes. The female reproductive system

- ☛ creates, releases, and transports the female reproductive cell. This cell is called an egg. The egg's job is to unite with a sperm cell. If it does not do this, it is absorbed by the body.
- ☛ provides a place for a baby to grow and develop before birth. It protects and nourishes this baby, which cannot yet survive on its own.
- ☛ delivers the newborn from the mother's body into the world.

A major purpose of the female reproductive system is to create egg cells. An egg cell is larger than a sperm cell. Each egg measures about $1/175$ of an inch. You can see an egg without a microscope, but it is only a tiny dot. A woman's ovaries produce

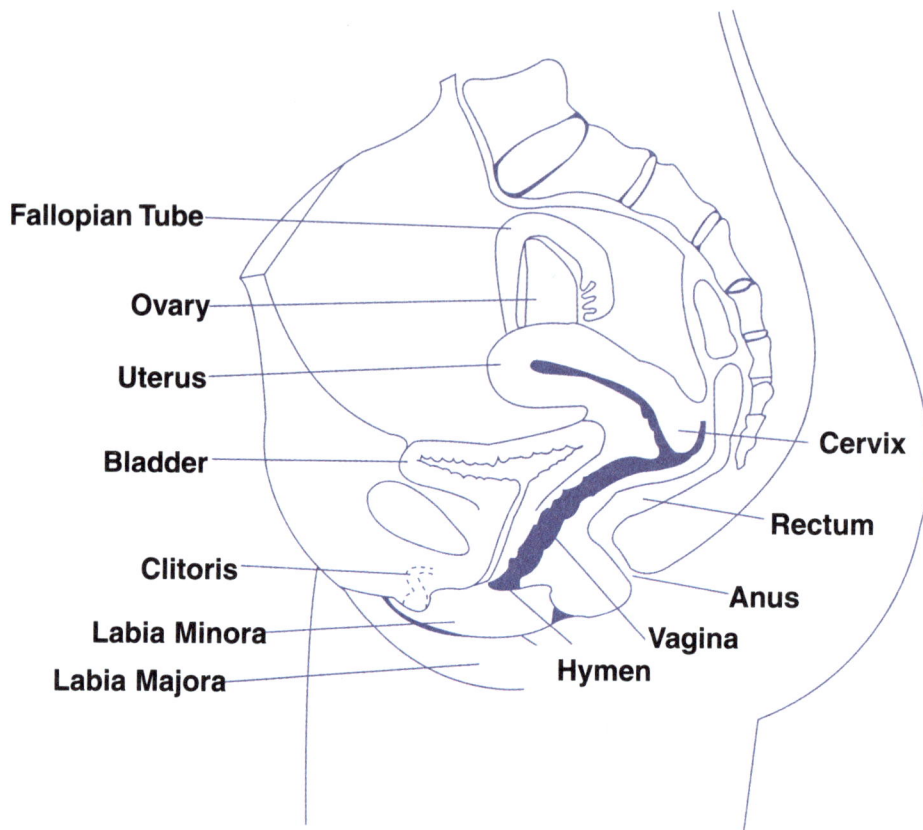

Fallopian Tube

Ovary

Uterus

Bladder

Clitoris

Labia Minora

Labia Majora

Cervix

Rectum

Anus

Vagina

Hymen

1-3 This side view of the female reproductive organs gives you an idea how they fit together inside the body.

and store eggs. Each ovary is small—about the size and shape of an almond. A female is born with about 400,000 eggs in her two ovaries. She will never make more. Her eggs do not begin to mature until puberty. A second job of the ovaries is to produce hormones. Each hormone plays a special role in the reproductive system.

Each month an ovary releases an egg. This egg travels through the reproductive system. See Figure 1-4. As it travels, the egg can be fertilized (united with a sperm). This is the time when pregnancy can occur. The egg keeps moving through the system until it is fertilized by a sperm or is absorbed by the body.

When an egg is released, it is drawn into the nearby fallopian tube. The fallopian (fuh-LOH-pee-uhn) tubes are two tubes in which eggs travel from the ovary to the uterus. Each fallopian tube has

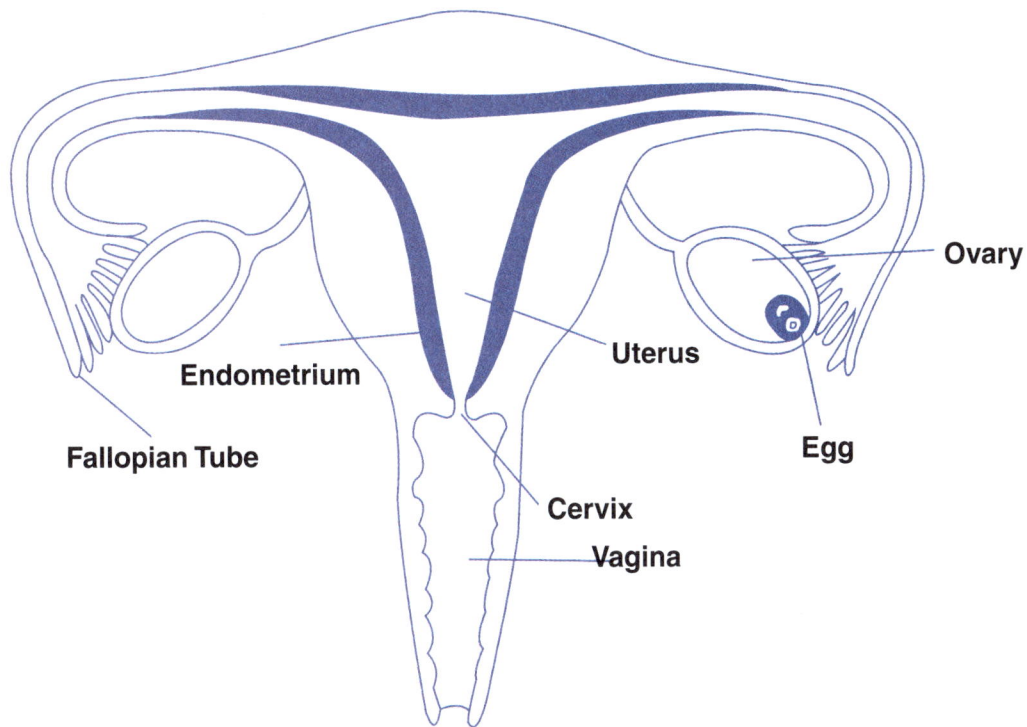

Ovary

Endometrium

Uterus

Fallopian Tube

Egg

Cervix

Vagina

1-4 Look at the egg and trace its path from the ovary to the outside of the body.

an open end near an ovary. This open end has fringes that can sweep the egg inside. The other end of the fallopian tube is attached to the uterus. The union of egg and sperm most often occurs inside a fallopian tube. If fertilized, the egg will travel into the uterus and implant there. If not, the egg will pass through the tube, into the uterus, and will be absorbed by the body.

The uterus (YOO-tuhr-uhs) is a muscular organ where a baby grows until birth. The uterus is sometimes called the womb (WOOM). It is found just behind the pubic bone. Picture an upside-down pear. This is the normal shape and size of the uterus. It also has a small, hollow space in the middle. The uterus has a spongy lining called the endometrium (ehn-doh-MEE-tree-uhm). During pregnancy, the fertilized egg will implant there. The uterus will stretch to the size of a watermelon to hold the growing baby. After the birth, the uterus slowly shrinks to its normal size.

The uterus has a small opening at the bottom. This narrow, muscular opening is called the cervix (SUR-vihks). When a woman is not pregnant, the cervix is thick and tight. Sperm enter the uterus through the cervix, and menstrual flow leaves through it. The penis does not enter the cervix during sexual intercourse. When a woman is pregnant, the cervix holds the growing baby inside the uterus. During childbirth, the cervix will stretch to allow the baby to pass through. After delivery, the cervix will return to its normal size. Your cervix is tested for cancer when you have a Pap smear. It does not hurt when you touch the cervix. It feels firm, much like the tip of your nose.

The cervix connects to the vagina (vuh-JY-nuh), a collapsed tube that extends from the cervix to the outside of the body. The vagina is also known as the birth canal. This muscular tunnel is about 4 to 5 inches long. It stretches like a rubber band during sexual intercourse to allow the penis to enter. It also stretches during childbirth. The vaginal opening can be seen on the outside of the female's body.

The opening of the vagina is part of the vulva. The vulva is the group of a woman's external reproductive organs. See Figure 1-5. The vulva has the following parts:

- ☞ The pubic mound is a fatty pad of tissue in front of the pubic bone. It is covered by pubic hair. The pubic mound protects and cushions the pubic region.
- ☞ The labia are two liplike flaps of skin near the vaginal opening. The outer lips are called the labia majora (LAY-bee-uh muh-JOH-ruh). The labia majora are covered with pubic hair. The hairless inner lips are called the labia minora (LAY-bee-uh muh-NOH-ruh). Both sets of labia protect the vagina and urinary opening.
- ☞ The clitoris (KLIH-tuhr-uhs) is a small, sensitive organ. It is found where the inner labia meet, just under the pubic hair. The clitoris has many nerve endings. Touching or rubbing the clitoris creates a pleasant sensation called sexual arousal. The peak of this sexual arousal is called an orgasm.

In Figure 1-4, you can see another opening—the urinary opening. It is located between the clitoris and vaginal opening. Urine leaves the body here. The opening is at the end of the urethra. The urethra is a long tube that carries urine from the bladder to the outside of

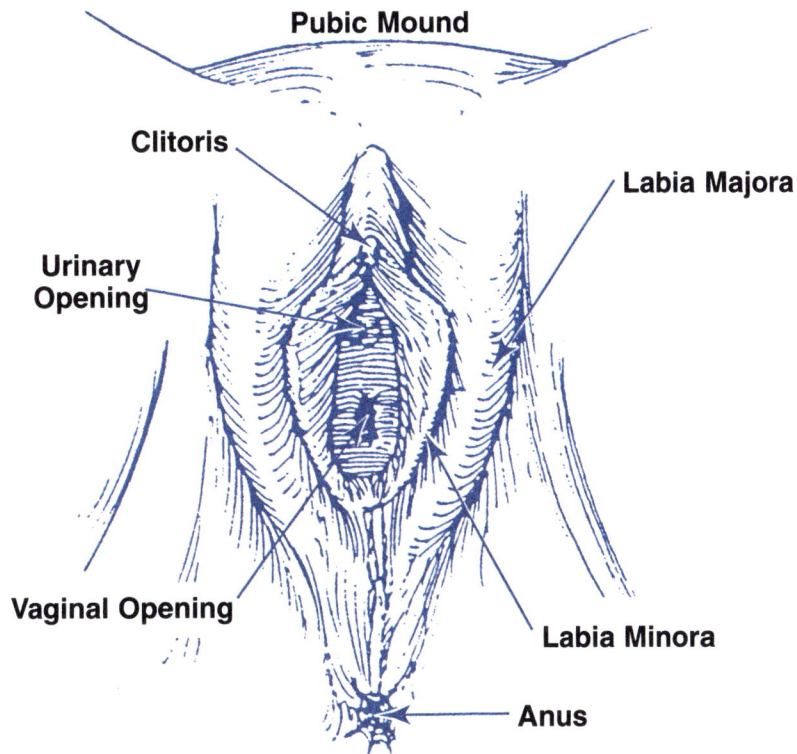

Pubic Mound

Clitoris

Urinary Opening

Labia Majora

Vaginal Opening

Labia Minora

Anus

1-5 The vulva is the name for the external parts of the female reproductive system.

the body. The female's urethra and urinary opening are not parts of her reproductive system. For this reason, they are not parts of the vulva. (The male's urethra is a part of his reproductive system.) It is helpful to know where these parts are, though, and what they do.

Now you have learned the major parts of the female reproductive system. Return to Figure 1-3 and Figure 1-4. Trace the path of the egg again and name each part of the system. Also, read the next section, which describes the menstrual cycle. This cycle plays a vital role in reproduction.

The Menstrual Cycle

The menstrual (MEHN-stroo-uhl) cycle is a series of monthly body changes in females. It prepares the body for a possible pregnancy. A girl's menstrual cycle will begin during puberty.

The ovaries receive a signal from the brain to begin making more female hormones and ripen an egg. In most young women, this happens at about age 12. It may also start as early as 9 or as late as age 16.

The menstrual cycle has two parts—ovulation and menstruation. See Figure 1-6. During ovulation (ahv-YUH-lay-shun), an ovary releases a mature egg. The egg is drawn into the fallopian tube. Here, it can unite with a sperm. At this time (mid-cycle), pregnancy is most likely to occur.

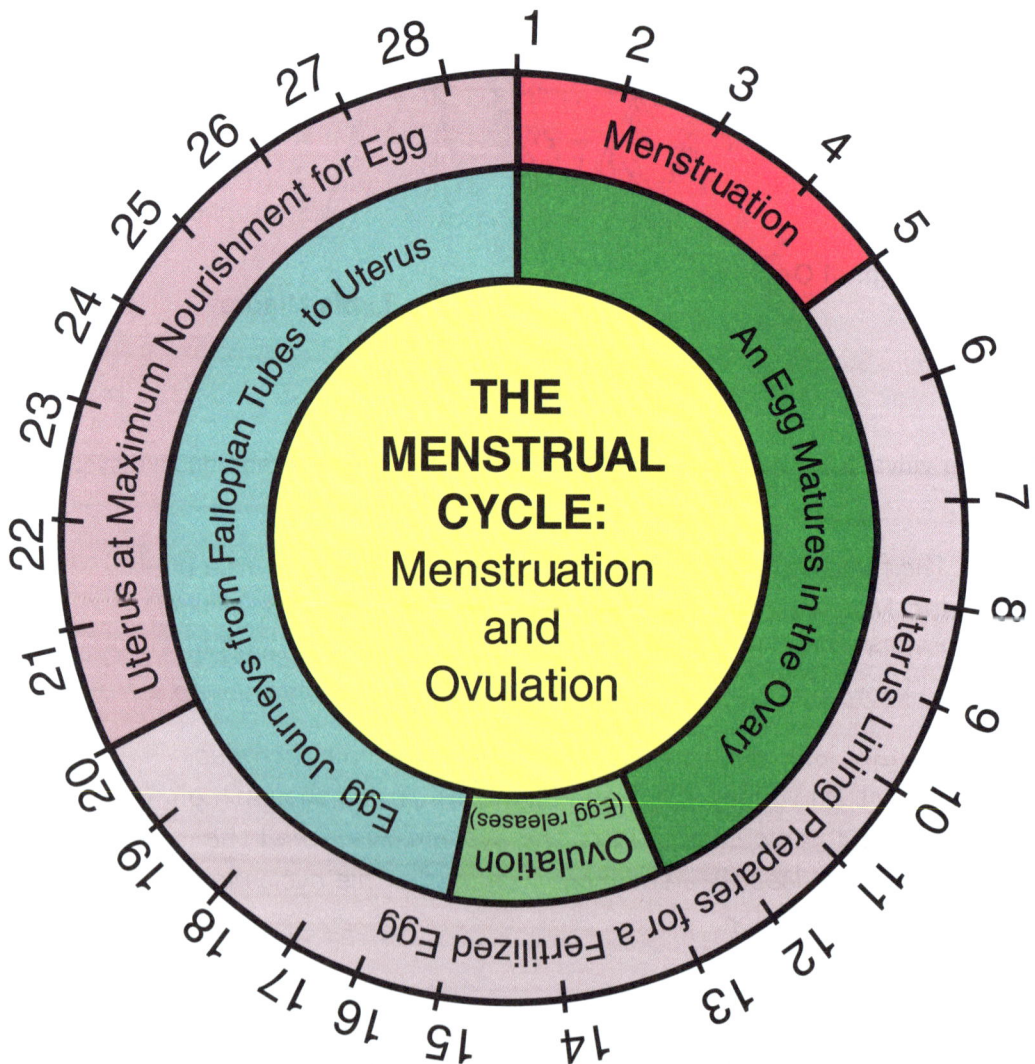

THE MENSTRUAL CYCLE: Menstruation and Ovulation

Menstruation

An Egg Matures in the Ovary

Uterus Lining Prepares for a Fertilized Egg

Ovulation (Egg releases)

Egg Journeys from Fallopian Tubes to Uterus

Uterus at Maximum Nourishment for Egg

1-6 A woman's menstrual cycle begins again about every 28 days. In most women, this process provides a mature egg each cycle that can be fertilized.

Hormones help the body prepare for pregnancy. They do this by thickening the endometrium. This thick lining of the uterus is rich in extra blood and other tissues. The body will need these tissues if pregnancy occurs. A fertilized egg can implant here. The thickened lining will provide nourishment for the growing baby.

If pregnancy does not happen, the lining is not needed. The extra blood and tissues leave the body during menstruation (men-stroo-WAY-shun). A woman might refer to menstruation as her menstrual period or just her period. Menstruation occurs once during each menstrual cycle.

One menstrual cycle lasts from the first day of a period to the first day of the next period. The first day of a period is day 1. Ovulation usually occurs around day 14, or halfway through the cycle. It can happen at any time in the cycle, though. A new menstrual cycle begins on the first day of the next period.

The average menstrual cycle is 28 days long. It is also normal for it to range from 21 days to 35 days. This can vary a great deal. Teens often have less regular cycles because their bodies are just getting used to this process. Menstrual cycles can also be affected by diet, stress, weight change, and extreme amounts of exercise.

Conception: The Beginning of Pregnancy

The creation of new life is one of the wonders of nature. Two tiny cells come together to become one. Over nine months, this single cell grows into a baby. This process begins with an event called conception. Conception is the union of an egg and sperm cell. Another name for this event is fertilization.

The Meeting of the Egg and Sperm

To make a baby, egg and sperm must combine in the female's body. Most of the time, this happens when the male delivers sperm to the female through ejaculation during sexual intercourse. In a single ejaculation, about two to three teaspoons of semen is released. It contains anywhere from 100 to 400 million sperm.

These sperm swim very quickly through the vagina, cervix, uterus, and fallopian tubes. Their mission is to find and penetrate the egg. It takes only one sperm to cause pregnancy!

Sperm can also enter the body even if ejaculation does not occur. Even before ejaculation, the penis can release a small amount of fluid called pre-ejaculatory fluid. This fluid has a high concentration of sperm. A woman could easily conceive from the sperm in this fluid. This is what makes withdrawing the penis from the vagina before ejaculation such an unreliable way to prevent pregnancy.

Once sperm enter the female's body, they can live for up to three days. (Some studies suggest sperm may live even longer.) An egg is fertile for about a day. If a fertile egg and a live sperm are present at the same time, conception can occur. This almost always happens in the fallopian tubes. Conception can happen the day intercourse occurs or a few days later. See Figure 1-7.

More than 100 sperm may reach the egg, but only one can enter. The sperm secrete a chemical to weaken the coating of the egg. Finally, one sperm works its way through. At this instant, the egg sends out a short electrical shock to keep the other sperm out. A hard coating forms to protect the egg that has now been fertilized. This fertilized egg forms a single cell called a zygote (ZY-goht). The zygote contains all the information needed to grow into a baby.

At once, this zygote begins to grow. Within hours of conception, the zygote divides into two cells that are exactly the same. The two cells divide into four, the four into eight, and so on. This division of each cell continues. The growing mass of cells clumps together in a ball shape.

Implantation in the Uterus

In most pregnancies, this growing ball of cells moves through the fallopian tube and into the uterus. This journey takes about 5 days. When it gets to the uterus, the ball contains about 100 to 150 cells. In the uterus, the ball of cells will attach to the endometrium. This is called implantation. Implantation is complete

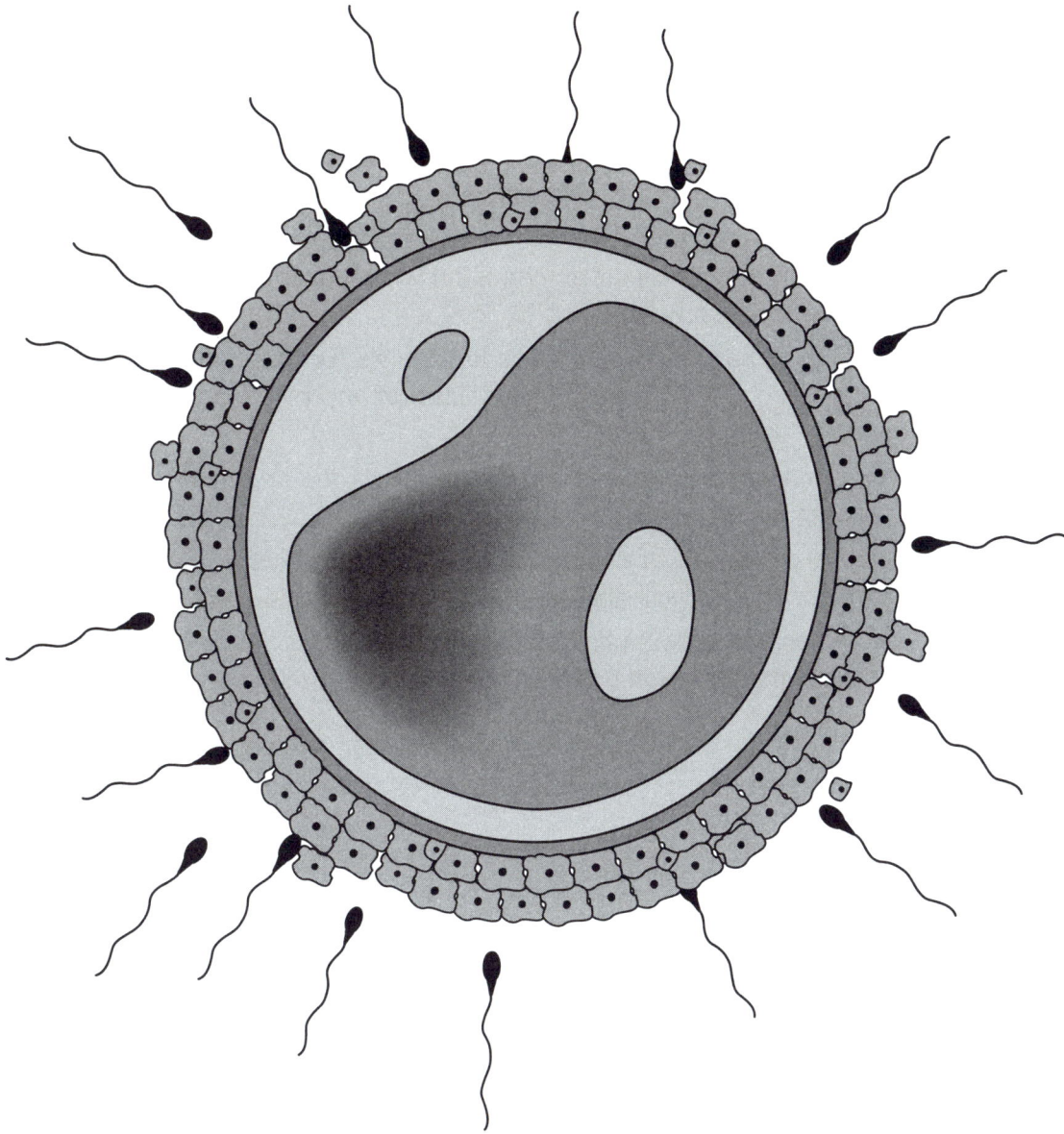

1-7 Many sperm try to penetrate the egg, but only one is allowed to enter.

within 10 to 12 days after conception. The baby will remain attached in the uterus as it grows. The rich lining will nourish the baby. The woman is pregnant, but she probably doesn't know it yet. Soon, however, she will learn of the pregnancy.

Major Points

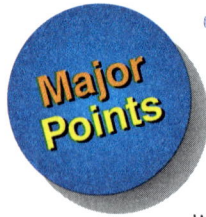

☞ Learning about the male and female reproductive systems can help you better understand how pregnancy occurs.

☞ The male reproductive system is responsible for creating sperm cells and delivering them to the woman's egg cell.

☞ The female reproductive system creates, releases, and transports egg cells. If an egg is fertilized, it will attach and grow in the woman's body.

☞ The menstrual cycle makes it possible for pregnancy to happen. It releases mature eggs for fertilization and builds a lining on the endometrium.

☞ Conception (fertilization) occurs when one sperm penetrates the egg. It is the beginning of pregnancy.

☞ As the result of conception, a single cell called a zygote is formed. This cell will grow and divide as it travels toward the uterus.

☞ When the growing ball of cells embeds itself in the lining of the uterus, implantation occurs.

Chapter 2 Confirming a Pregnancy

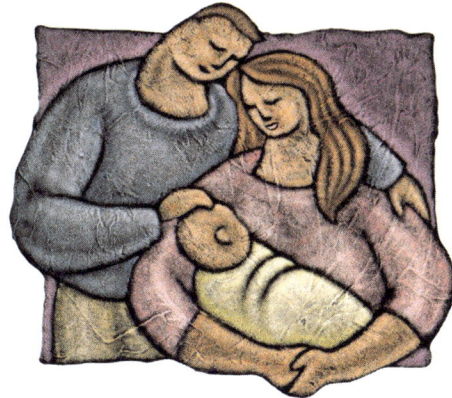

No signs or symptoms tell a woman conception has occurred. She cannot yet feel the changes going on in her body. It may be several weeks before she notices any changes. When she does, she might begin to suspect she is pregnant. Knowing the early signs of pregnancy is helpful. It can make it easier for a woman to know when she might be pregnant. This way she can seek testing right away. This is best for her and her baby, if she is indeed pregnant.

Early Signs of Pregnancy

Several common signs are linked to pregnancy. By itself, none of these signs is a guarantee. Each sign can occur for reasons other than pregnancy. A woman may notice only one sign or many of them. A few women don't have any early signs. If you think you might be pregnant, you should have a pregnancy test done.

A missed or late period is often the first sign of pregnancy. Many teens do not notice this sign because their periods are not regular. You may not always know when to expect your period. Keeping track of your periods on a calendar will help. This way you can learn what is normal for you. Having a period that is not normal for you (too light, too early, or too late) can be a sign of pregnancy. Figure 2-1 shows other early signs of pregnancy.

Have you had one or more of these signs? Did you have sexual intercourse since your last normal period? If you answer yes to both questions, you may be pregnant. Have a test as soon as possible so you will know for sure. You might be scared to find out. Many teens say wondering is worse than knowing the truth.

Where to Go for Tests

Many teens have questions about pregnancy testing. You may have mixed feelings about the test. It can be helpful to talk with someone. Talk to an adult you trust. Parents are often the best choice. Even though they may be angry at first, most parents want to help their children. If you cannot ask your parents, maybe you can talk to a teacher, counselor, or school nurse. These adults may be able to answer questions and help you get a test.

If you do not have an adult you can talk with, you might talk to a friend or your partner. Your partner and friends may <u>not</u> have all the answers you need. They may not know much about pregnancy tests or where to get them. They can provide emotional support, though. It helps to have a friend with you.

Early Signs of Pregnancy

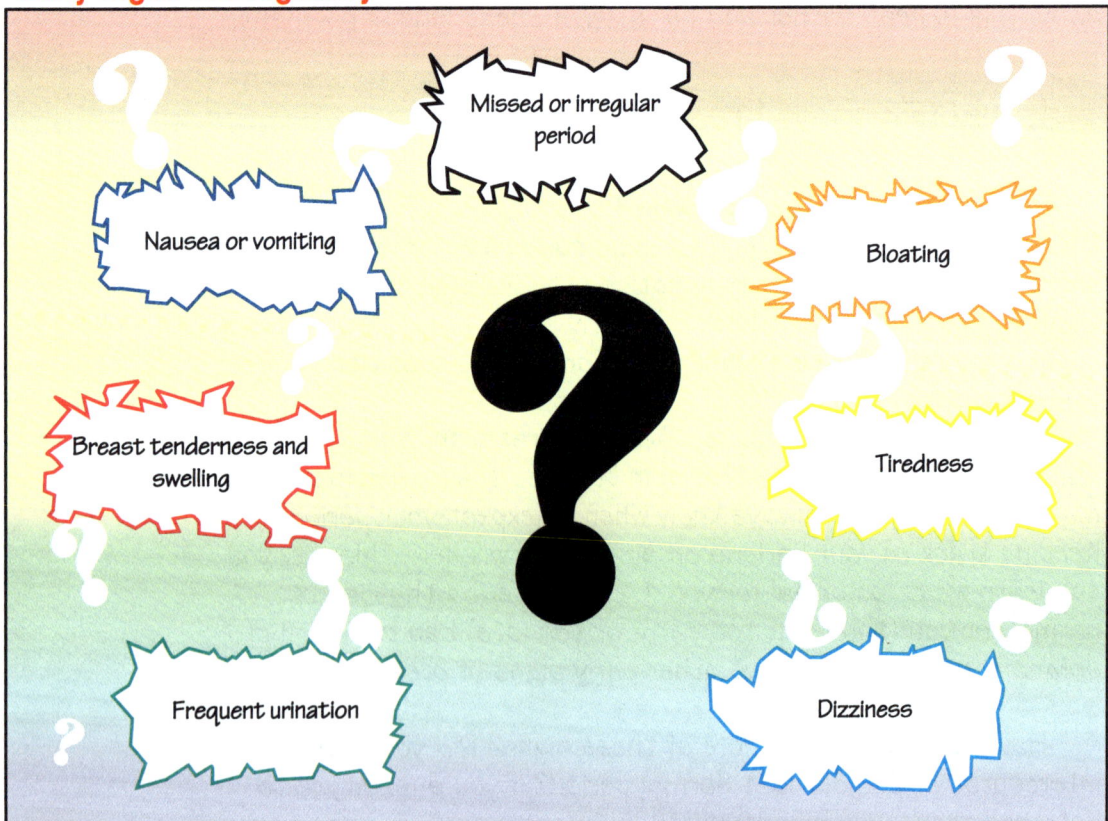

Missed or irregular period

Nausea or vomiting

Bloating

Breast tenderness and swelling

Tiredness

Frequent urination

Dizziness

2-1   What signs of pregnancy have you noticed (did you notice)?

Some teens choose to go for pregnancy testing alone. You can take the test by yourself. This option has a bad side, though. You will miss the support of those closest to you. It can be tough to go through this alone. If you do, try to find someone you can talk to afterward.

You may wonder where to go for a pregnancy test. There are a few options. Health care providers and pregnancy testing centers can help you. A third choice is a home pregnancy test.

Health Care Provider

Can you talk to your parents about the chance you might be pregnant? If so, they may want you to visit your regular health care provider for a test. A health care provider is a person or agency licensed to provide medical care. This is most often a doctor or clinic. Your health care provider knows you and your medical history. He or she can recommend the best care for you. If your parents have insurance for you, the office visit may be covered. Insurance may or may not pay for the test.

Tests done by professionals are the most accurate. You can find good care in a clinic, doctor's office, or hospital. If you're pregnant, your provider can tell you what medical care you will need. Your test can be the start of this care. If you're not pregnant, you can ask your provider about how to prevent pregnancy in the future.

Pregnancy Testing Center

What if you choose not to see a health care provider? You may not want to ask your family doctor for a test for some reason. You might not have insurance or want your parents' insurance to be billed. The test and office visit might cost too much. If these factors are an issue, search for other local services. Some towns and cities have pregnancy testing centers. These centers offer free or low-cost testing.

The tests might be anonymous. This means no one would know who you are. Instead, they might be confidential, which means you would have to give your name. Your results would still be kept private. Most centers also offer counseling and will refer you to other places in your area that can help.

You can find pregnancy testing centers in the phone book. They are often listed under <u>Pregnancy</u> or <u>Clinics</u>. Some centers are run by churches or other groups. If this matters to you, call and ask. You should also call ahead with any questions you have about the center's services.

Home Pregnancy Test

A third option is a home pregnancy test. You can buy this type of test in a drugstore or supermarket. A home pregnancy test can be fairly accurate. A home test can give you privacy. Some women prefer to take this type of test before going to see their health care providers. If your test is positive, see your provider as soon as possible.

Before you use a home pregnancy test, read the directions carefully. You must follow them exactly. A single mistake could affect the results. If you have questions, call the toll-free number on the instruction sheet (if one is given). You can also call a health care provider. A nurse can answer your questions.

If your test result is negative, you are probably not pregnant. However, you may have taken the test too soon to tell for sure. Take another test a week or two later if you still think you might be pregnant. If you still wonder after your second test, visit a health care provider. If you're not pregnant, you may feel happy and relieved. You might also feel a little sad. This is normal. Use this time to focus on preventing pregnancy until you are ready.

The Next Steps If You Are Pregnant

What if your pregnancy test comes out positive? What should you do next? You have many big decisions to make and a lot to do. At first, these responsibilities may overwhelm you. See Figure 2-2. Try to take things one step at a time. You do not have to figure everything out at once. There are only a few steps you must take right now.

Get Medical Care

When you are pregnant, your first and most important step is to get medical care. Your health care provider can tell how far along you are in your pregnancy. This person can figure out when your baby is due. This is true even if you're not sure when your last period started. He or she can make sure you and your baby are healthy. Your health care provider will test for infections and conditions that might harm the baby. He or she can also refer you to a counselor if you need help sorting out your feelings about the pregnancy.

Early medical care can prevent some health problems. If problems do exist, they can be treated right away. Early medical care can help you make good health choices. These choices will protect you and your baby. Your baby will be less likely to be born too early, too small, or both. He will be less likely to have serious medical problems.

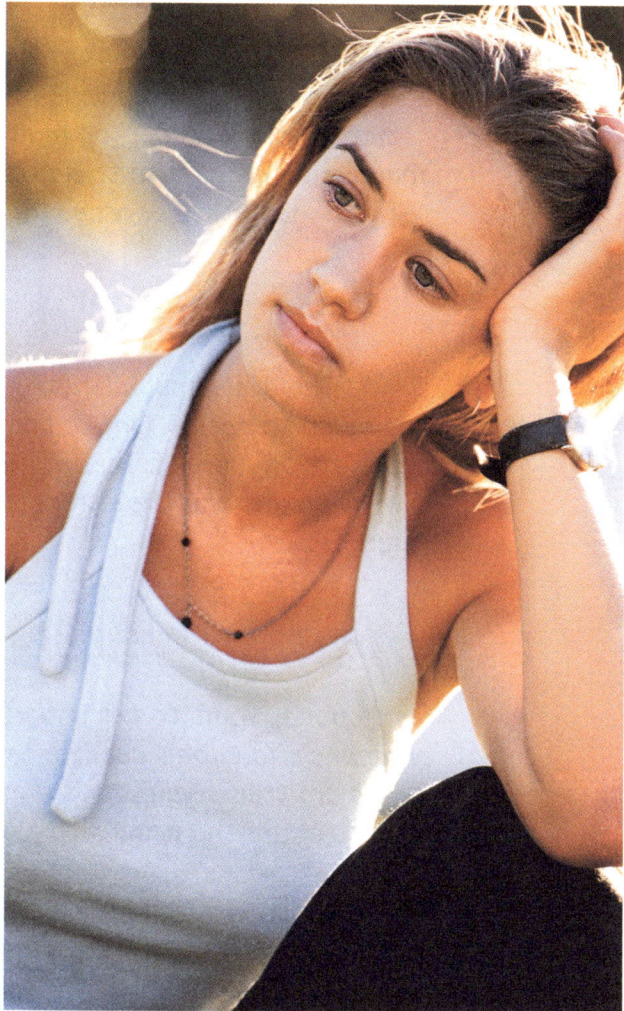

2-2 Knowing you're pregnant brings a lot to think about. Be patient with yourself and your mixed emotions, though.

If you have started human papillomavirus (HPV) vaccine series of injections, it is better to continue the series after your pregnancy. This vaccine protects you against cancers of the cervix, vulva, and vagina.

What if you don't have health insurance? Try a health department, hospital, or clinic. Talk to a social worker or financial counselor there. This person will know what services are available. Many places offer free or low-cost services. In some states, a teen can apply for pregnancy health insurance. Your town or city may offer special medical care just for pregnant teens. If so, a school nurse or counselor can tell you about it. You can also look in the phone book under Pregnancy.

You might also call your local public aid office. It should be listed in the phone book. You may qualify for Medicaid. This government program provides free medical care to those who cannot afford it. A person must meet certain guidelines to apply. You might also be able to get other public aid. A caseworker can tell you what other services in your area might be helpful.

Take Care of Yourself

At this time, much is going on in your life. You have much to do and much to decide. One of the best things you can do right now is take care of yourself. This will help you and your baby stay healthy. It will also give you the strength to face the challenges ahead. See Figure 2-3.

Tell Important People

You may want to tell important people in your life about the pregnancy. You don't need to tell everyone right now, though. This is even more true if you aren't sure yet what you will do. It may be best to share the news with just a few people right now.

Most likely, your partner is one of the first people you should tell. He helped create the pregnancy. He needs to know you are pregnant. You're carrying the baby, but your partner's also involved. He has rights and responsibilities when it comes to the baby.

Taking Care of Yourself

❖ Get plenty of sleep and exercise.

❖ Eat nutritious foods.

❖ Spend some time every day relaxing.

❖ Avoid dangerous substances, such as alcohol, tobacco, and other drugs.

❖ Seek medical care.

2-3 Following these guidelines will help you feel your best.

In some situations, telling the baby's father may be tough. The two of you may not be together anymore. You may not get along well. You may not want to have a relationship. He is still the father of your baby, though. If you have serious concerns about telling him, talk with a trusted adult about it. In a few cases, it might be safer <u>not</u> to tell him.

Just as important is deciding when to tell your family. You may wonder which family members to tell and when to tell them. It might worry you how they will react. You might feel afraid about what they will do and say. You may wonder about how to tell them. Many parents will be angry at first. They may need some time to adjust to the idea. In time, many parents can understand and be supportive.

Some teens feel they cannot tell their parents. They may think they don't need their parents' help or permission to get prenatal care. This may or may not be true. It depends on the policies of health care providers in your area. If you continue the pregnancy, it's not realistic to think your parents will never know! One day, your pregnancy will show.

Many mothers are very aware of the early signs of pregnancy. Your mother may suspect you are pregnant even before you do! Some teens want help telling their parents the news. If so, maybe you can ask an older sister, aunt, or grandmother to help. You might also ask a close family friend or someone from your house of worship.

Find the Support You Need

Your family may be very supportive of you. Some pregnant teens are surprised how well their families react. Other families don't handle the news as well. They might disown the pregnant teen and ask her to leave their home. How was your relationship with your family before you were pregnant? This is often the best predictor of what it will be like in the future.

Your friends or partner might be the easiest ones to talk to about your pregnancy. See Figure 2-4. On the other hand, you might lose friends or have your partner leave you because of the pregnancy. It is hard to tell in advance what will

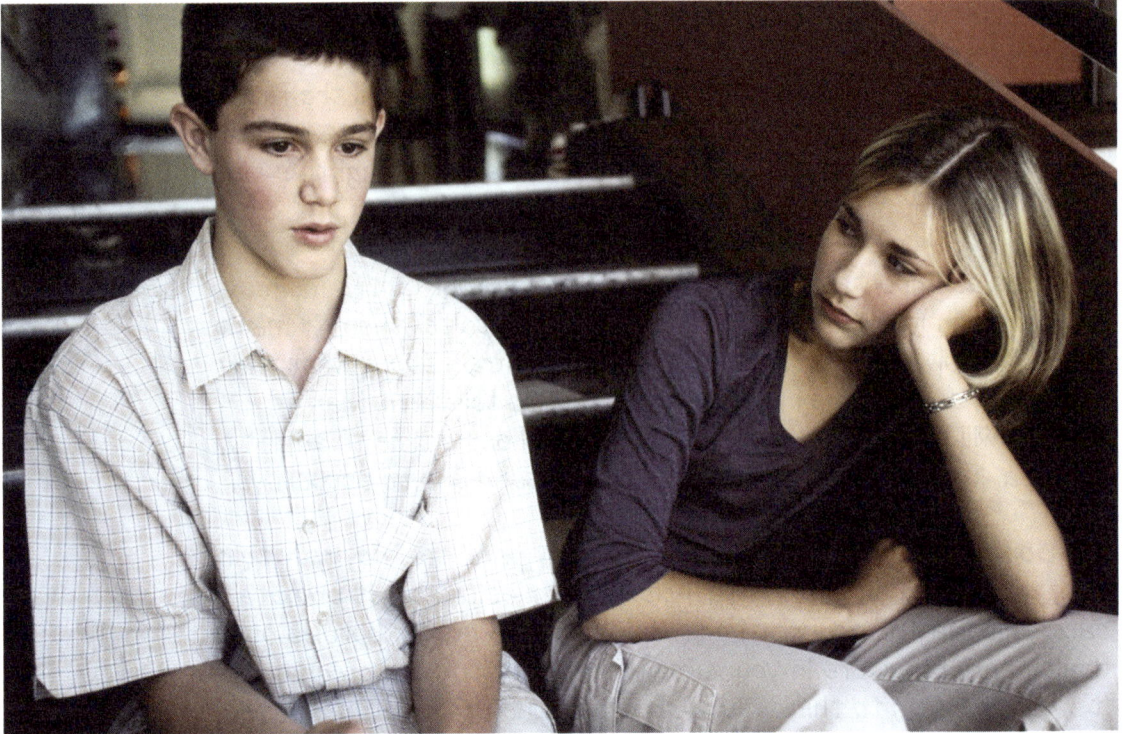

2-4 You and your partner have a lot to talk about regarding the pregnancy. It will provide tremendous support if the two of you can go through this together.

happen. Each person's situation is different. At this time, you will quickly learn who supports you even when things are difficult. These are the people you can rely on to help you.

What if you don't get enough support from family, friends, and your partner? Look to your community. Can you talk to a teacher, nurse, or counselor at school? Is there a professional counselor, social worker, or therapist you can talk with? Such a person is well trained to help with these matters. He or she might even be able to help you tell your parents.

Talk to your support person about your thoughts and feelings. As you begin to make decisions, talk them through with this person. Your support person should <u>not</u> tell you what choice to make. Instead, he or she should listen and help you clarify your options and goals.

Start Learning About Your Options

Now that you're pregnant, you have many decisions to make. Will you give birth? Will you parent your child or make an adoption plan? Where will you live? How will you stay in school? Will you work? You don't need to make all these decisions at once. In fact, it's better not to rush such important decisions. Take your time to arrive at the best choices for you and your baby.

Right now, you can begin by learning about your options. Professionals can answer many of your questions. Talking with your family and partner may show you options you haven't considered. Ask your school nurse about agencies that can help you. Being informed can help you make good decisions.

Danger Signs of Early Pregnancy

Most pregnancies proceed without any problems. However, it is important to watch for danger signs. These signs could mean the health of you and your baby are at risk. You can reduce your risk by knowing the danger signs. If you notice any of these, call your health care provider right away. See Figure 2-5.

Ectopic Pregnancy

When an egg is fertilized, it should move toward the uterus. It should attach there and grow. In some cases, the fertilized egg will attach and grow in the wrong place. This is

Danger Signs

Contact your health care provider at once if you notice any of the following:

* severe abdominal or pelvic pain
* cramping
* vaginal bleeding
* inability to keep foods or liquids in your stomach

* painful urination
* burning sensation during urination

2-5 If you notice any of these danger signs, call your health care provider right away.

called an ectopic (ehk-TAH-pihk) pregnancy. It can be very dangerous for the woman. About 100,000 ectopic pregnancies occur each year in the United States.

In most of these pregnancies, the fertilized egg stays in the fallopian tube and begins to grow there. (This is sometimes called a tubal pregnancy.) The fallopian tube is small and doesn't stretch much. A growing embryo can cause the fallopian tube to burst. This can cause a woman to bleed heavily. It can also lower her chances of pregnancy in the future. The fallopian tubes are needed for conception. If one bursts, the woman's chances to get pregnant in the future will be reduced. <u>An ectopic pregnancy is a medical emergency!</u>

Ectopic pregnancy can occur for many reasons. In teens, it is often linked to pelvic inflammatory disease (PID). With PID, the female reproductive organs can become infected and inflamed. PID can scar the fallopian tubes. This scar tissue can prevent a fertilized egg from moving to the uterus. The egg is more likely to attach and grow in the tubes. PID is most often caused by sexually transmitted infections (STIs).

Severe pain in the lower abdominal or pelvic area is the major sign of ectopic pregnancy. This pain is usually located on one side. Other signs are cramping and a missed or unusual period (early, late, lighter flow, or spotting).

If you think you might have an ectopic pregnancy, seek help at once! Go to your health care provider or the emergency room. You will need a pregnancy test and examination. In an ectopic pregnancy, surgery may be needed. The affected tube may have to be removed. Sometimes a strong medicine can be used to avoid surgery.

Miscarriage

Miscarriage is the body's way to end a pregnancy before its fifth month. This happens most often in the first trimester. It is usually not known why miscarriage occurs. Problems with the growing baby are the most common reason.

Other factors linked to a high risk of miscarriage are the following:

- ☛ mother's use of alcohol, tobacco, or drugs
- ☛ lack of health care early in pregnancy
- ☛ infections or untreated STIs in the mother

Cramping, pelvic pain, and bleeding can be signs of a miscarriage. Once a woman has begun to miscarry, little can be done to stop it. If you have these symptoms, call your health care provider right away. Your provider can find out for sure what is happening. Health care can also reduce the risk of further problems.

Dehydration

Both you and your growing baby need lots of fluids. Water and other fluids are vital to the body. If you don't have enough fluids, it can harm you and your baby. Dehydration means the body's fluid level is too low.

Early in pregnancy this can be a serious concern. At this time, nausea and vomiting are common. Fluids are often lost through vomiting. You are at risk for dehydration if you can't keep any food or liquid in your stomach for 24 hours. If this happens, call your health care provider. You may need to take fluids intravenously (by IV). This will restore your body's fluid level.

Urinary Tract Infections

A woman should watch for signs of urinary tract infection (UTI). This happens most often in the early months of pregnancy. A UTI infects the kidneys, bladder, and urethra. Symptoms of a UTI include the following:

- ☛ painful urination
- ☛ burning sensation when you urinate
- ☛ frequent urination

Call your health care provider if you have these symptoms. Your provider can tell you whether you have a urinary tract infection. If so, he or she will know how to treat it.

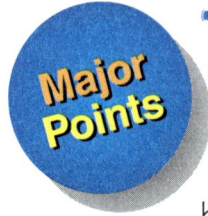

Major Points

☞ A missed or irregular period is often the first sign of pregnancy. Other early signs can also occur.

☞ If you suspect you may be pregnant, you should be tested right away. You can choose a health care provider, pregnancy testing center, or home pregnancy test kit.

☞ During pregnancy, it is vital to seek early medical care and take care of yourself.

☞ Telling your partner and family about the pregnancy can be difficult. Parents or other family members are usually the best people to help you make decisions about your pregnancy.

☞ Finding the support you need can make it easier for you to start learning about your options.

☞ Early in pregnancy, you should watch for danger signs of ectopic pregnancy, miscarriage, dehydration, and urinary tract infection. Report any signs to your health care provider at once.

Chapter 3 Understanding Your Pregnancy

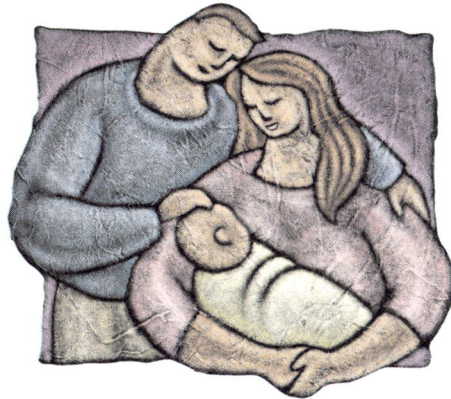

A pregnancy lasts just over nine months or about 40 weeks. It involves the bodies of two people—mother and baby. During this time, both experience a great deal of change. As the mother, you will see and feel many changes in your body and emotions. Your baby will start as one tiny cell and grow into an infant ready to be born.

This chapter describes how your baby will grow and change in the next few months. It also tells you what changes to expect in your own body. Some of the normal discomforts are explained, and tips are given for handling them. You will learn what emotional changes are common and how to cope with them.

A Boy or a Girl?

Most parents-to-be wonder if they will have a girl or boy. Some are eager to find out even before the baby is born. Other new parents want to be surprised at the birth. You may wonder about your baby's gender (sex). Nature has a special way to choose the gender of each infant.

A baby's gender depends on chromosomes. Chromosomes (KROH-muh-sohmz) are parts of cells that carry the traits that parents pass on to their children. The male's sperm has 23 chromosomes. The female's egg also has 23 chromosomes. During fertilization, these chromosomes combine in one cell called a zygote. The zygote has a total of 46 chromosomes—half from the mother and half from the father.

The chromosomes determine the traits a child will have. A few of these traits are skin, hair, and eye color. One set of chromosomes carries the trait for gender. It decides if the baby will be a boy or girl. The sex chromosome carried by the father's sperm determines a baby's gender.

Your Baby's Growth

Soon after conception, the zygote starts to grow and divide. Two types of cells are forming. One kind will become your baby's body. The other kind will make her support system. The main part of this system is the placenta. The placenta (pluh-SEHN-tuh) serves as an exchange site between the mother and baby. It develops against the wall of the uterus and looks like a flat piece of liver. Another part is the umbilical cord. The umbilical cord is a thick cord that contains three blood vessels. It connects the placenta to the baby's navel (belly button). The placenta and cord form her lifeline.

The mother's blood flows into the placenta. Her blood is full of food and oxygen, which is carried to the baby through the umbilical cord. The baby's blood flows through the umbilical cord to the placenta. It is full of waste products the baby doesn't need. This waste is picked up by the mother's blood and removed. Almost everything in the mother's blood can cross the placenta and reach the baby.

Surrounding the baby is a thin membrane called the amniotic (am-NEE-ah-tihk) sac. The amniotic sac protects the baby. It contains fluid in which she floats. For this reason, it is often called the bag of waters. The fluid is not water, though. Instead it is amniotic fluid. This fluid keeps the baby warm and gives her freedom to move. It also cushions her from injury and helps her to grow.

Month-by-Month Growth

It is amazing that a single cell can grow into a human being. This process takes time, though. That's why pregnancy lasts nine months. Each month, new and exciting changes occur. You can't see these changes, but they're happening inside you. A baby's growth and development before birth is called prenatal development. Knowing how your baby grows each month of pregnancy may make you feel closer to him.

The illustrations on the following pages show the progression of prenatal development. These images are close to actual size. The lengths and weights given are averages reached by the end of the month.

Month One
Length: ½ inch
Weight: less than an ounce

After implantation, the baby inside you is called an embryo (EHM-bree-oh). The embryo doesn't look much like a person at first. In fact, your baby has a tail that will later disappear! He lacks arms and legs, but does have limb buds. The major organs—the heart, lungs, brain, and spinal cord—are starting to take shape. Three and one-half weeks after conception, the heart starts beating. The placenta and the umbilical cord are forming.

Month Two
Length: 1 inch
Weight: a little less than an ounce

During the second month, the placenta begins working. It passes nutrients from you to your baby. It helps rid your baby's body of waste. The eyes, nose, ears, and mouth have begun to develop. His wrists and fingers are visible, as are ankles and weblike toes. Eyelids are forming but will be shut tight for a few more months. All the baby's internal organs and systems have started to develop. By the end of the second month, the embryo takes on a more human shape.

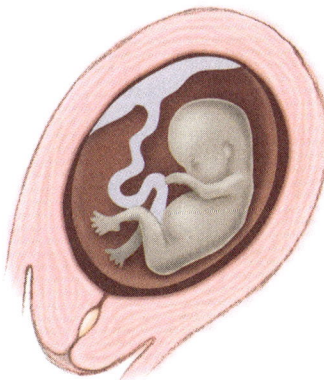

Month Three

Length: 4 inches

Weight: a little more than one ounce

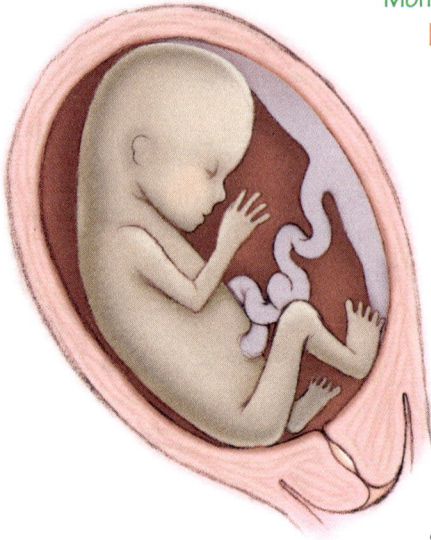

From the ninth week of pregnancy until birth, your baby is called a fetus (FEE-tihs). Soft fingernails and toenails are present. Inside the mouth, tiny buds are growing for the teeth, which will come in a few months after birth. By the end of this month, the baby's heartbeat is stronger. Your health care provider can use a special device to help you hear it. Many parents-to-be feel excited about this. Your baby's father or a support person might like to hear the heartbeat, too.

Month Four
Length: 6 to 7 inches
Weight: 5 ounces

During this month, the fetus begins to move more. The placenta has finished developing, but the umbilical cord is still growing. The external sex organs are now distinct. The baby's skin is pink and so thin you can see through it. His fingernails and toenails are growing. Late in this month, you may feel your baby move for the first time. The movements can't be felt from the outside of your abdomen yet, though. That will take about two more months.

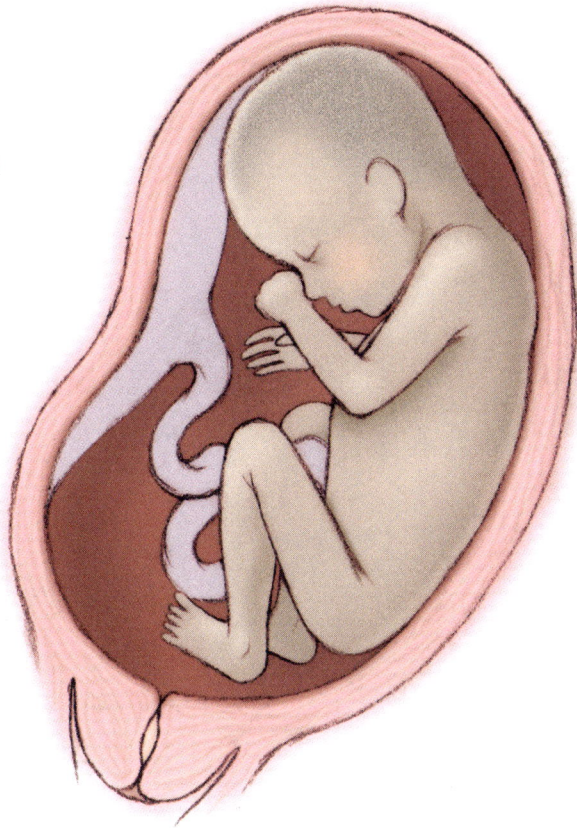

Month Five
Length: 8 to 12 inches
Weight: ½ to 1 pound

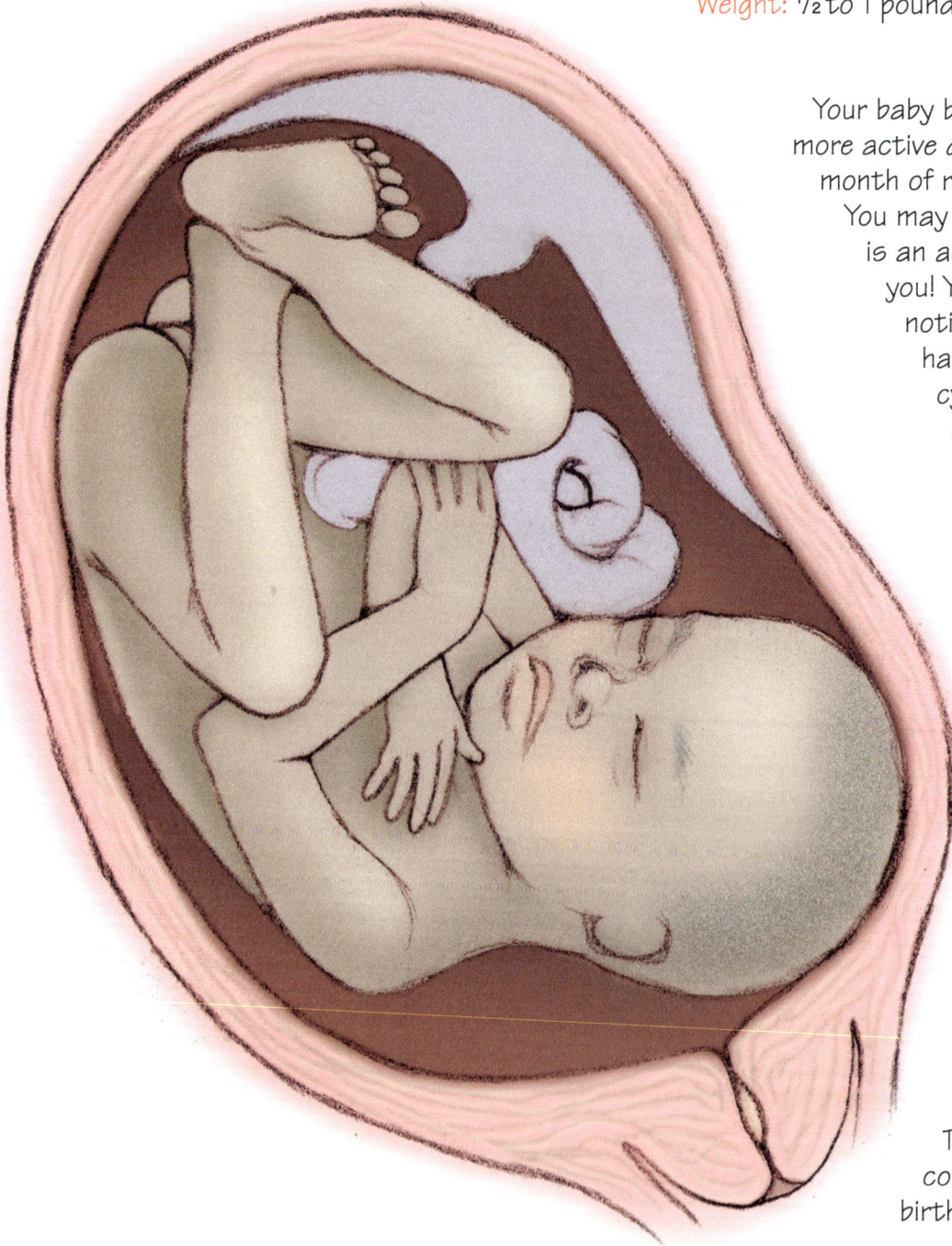

Your baby becomes even more active during this month of rapid growth. You may feel like there is an acrobat inside you! You will also notice your baby has his own sleep cycle. It is usually not the same as yours! Hair, eyelashes, and eyebrows grow. The brain develops a lot this month. Organs are continuing to grow and develop. The baby starts to grow quickly in size. This will continue until birth.

Month Six
Length: 11 to 14 inches
Weight: 1 to 1½ pounds

During the sixth month, the fetus kicks even harder and becomes even more active. Your baby has red, wrinkly skin. His skin is covered by a fine, soft hair called lanugo (luh-NOO-goh) and a white, waxy coating called vernix (VUR-nihks). The brain and body continue to grow at a fast pace. Finger- and toeprints are present. The eyelids begin to separate. Your baby can open his eyes. Babies born at the end of six months have a chance to survive. However, they need very special care in an intensive care unit.

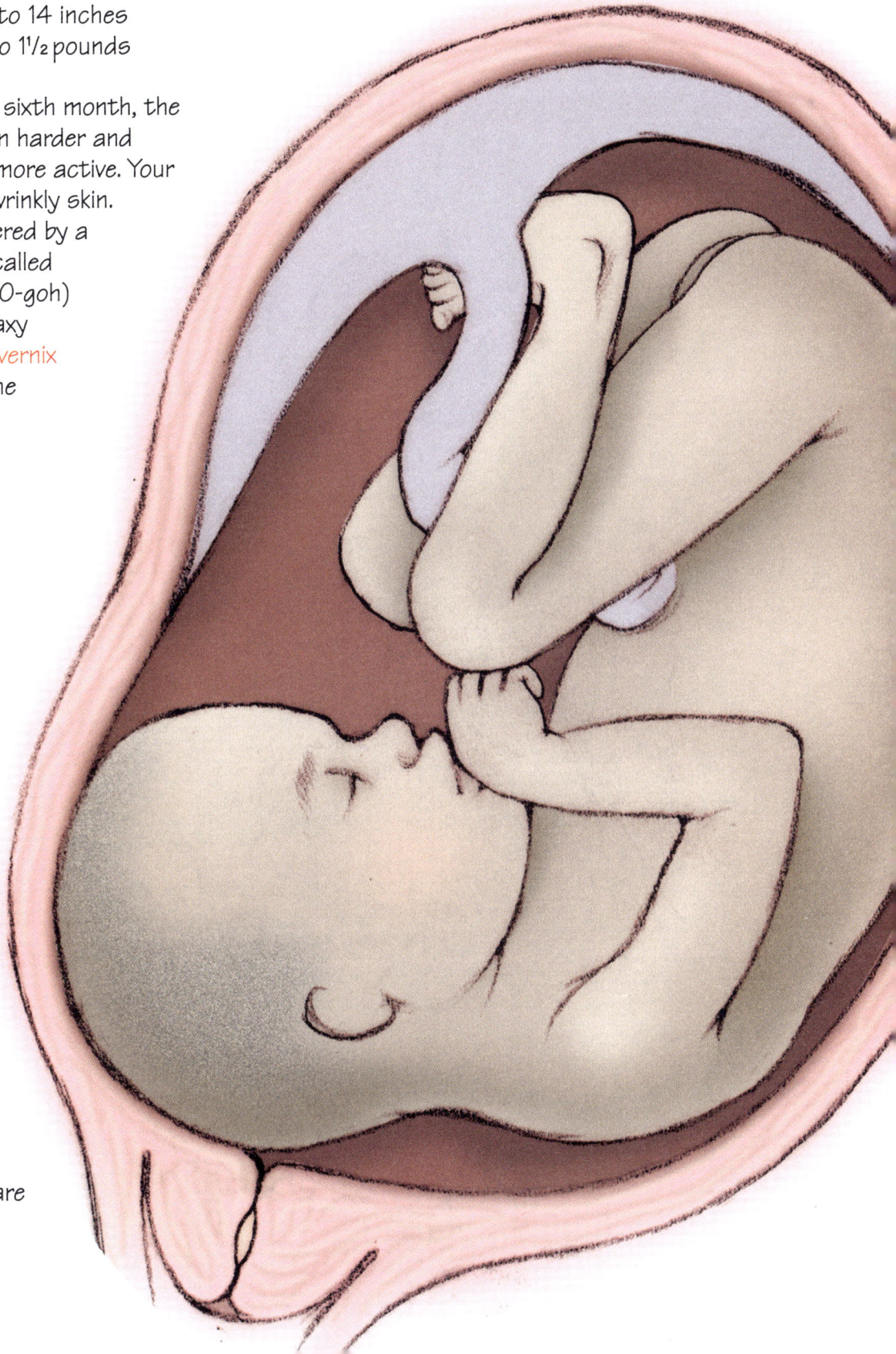

Month Seven
Length: 15 inches
Weight: 3 pounds

In this month, your baby's skin is less wrinkled. His body is adding fat stores to protect him against being cold outside the womb. Your baby can hear (and grow used to) your voice. You and the baby's father might sing or talk to him. He may find comfort in sucking his thumb. As the baby grows, there is less space in the uterus to move. That doesn't keep him from being active, though. Over half of all babies born in this month will survive. They do need special medical care, though.

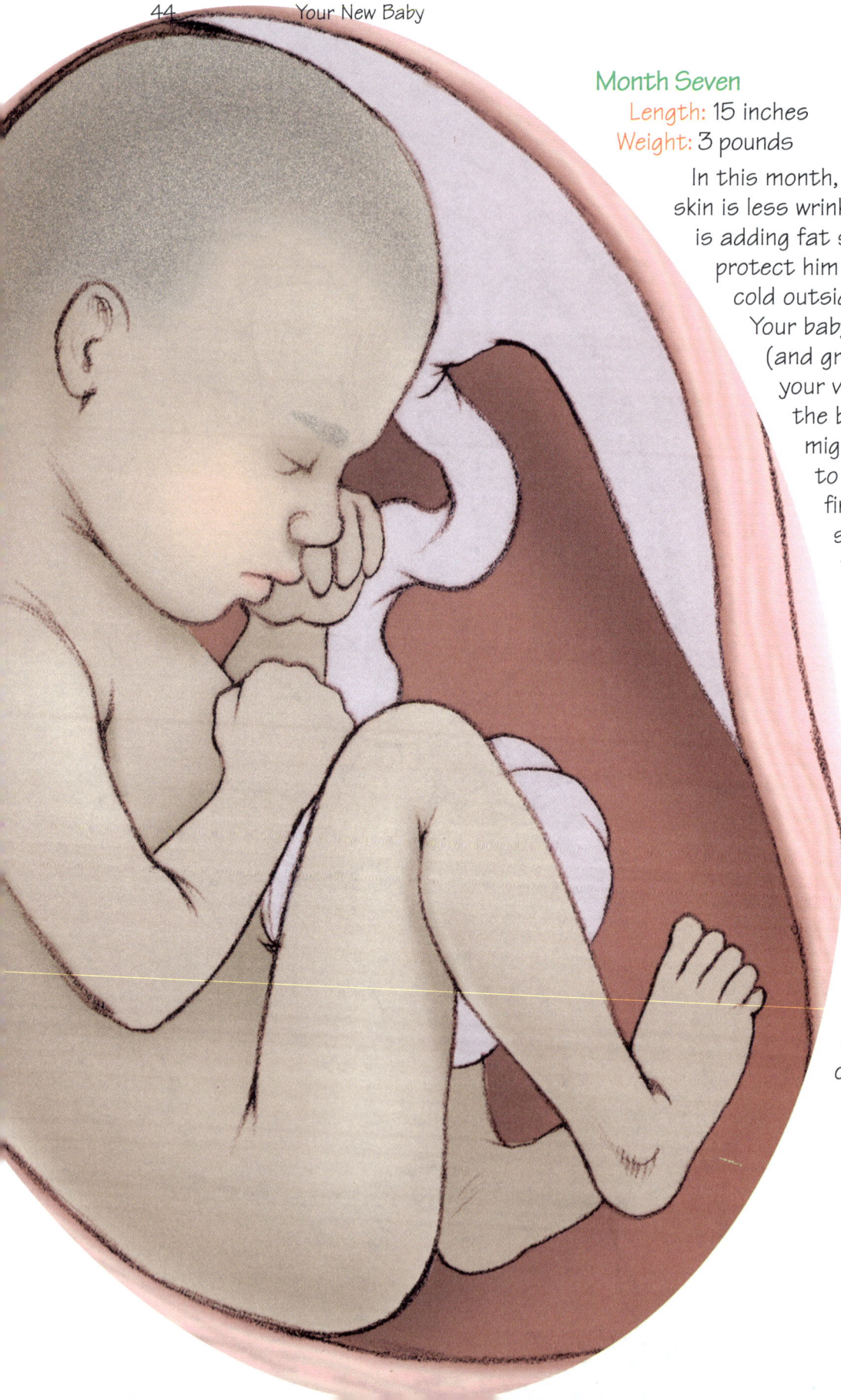

Month Eight
Length: 18 inches
Weight: 5 pounds

In the eighth month, the baby's brain keeps growing rapidly. His lungs are still immature. The bones are hard now, except those of the head. These bones are soft and flexible so the baby can fit through the birth canal. Your baby's kicks are stronger than before, but there is even less room for him to move. Sometimes you will notice the shape of an elbow or a foot poking up through your abdomen. Most babies born in the eighth month have a very good chance to survive.

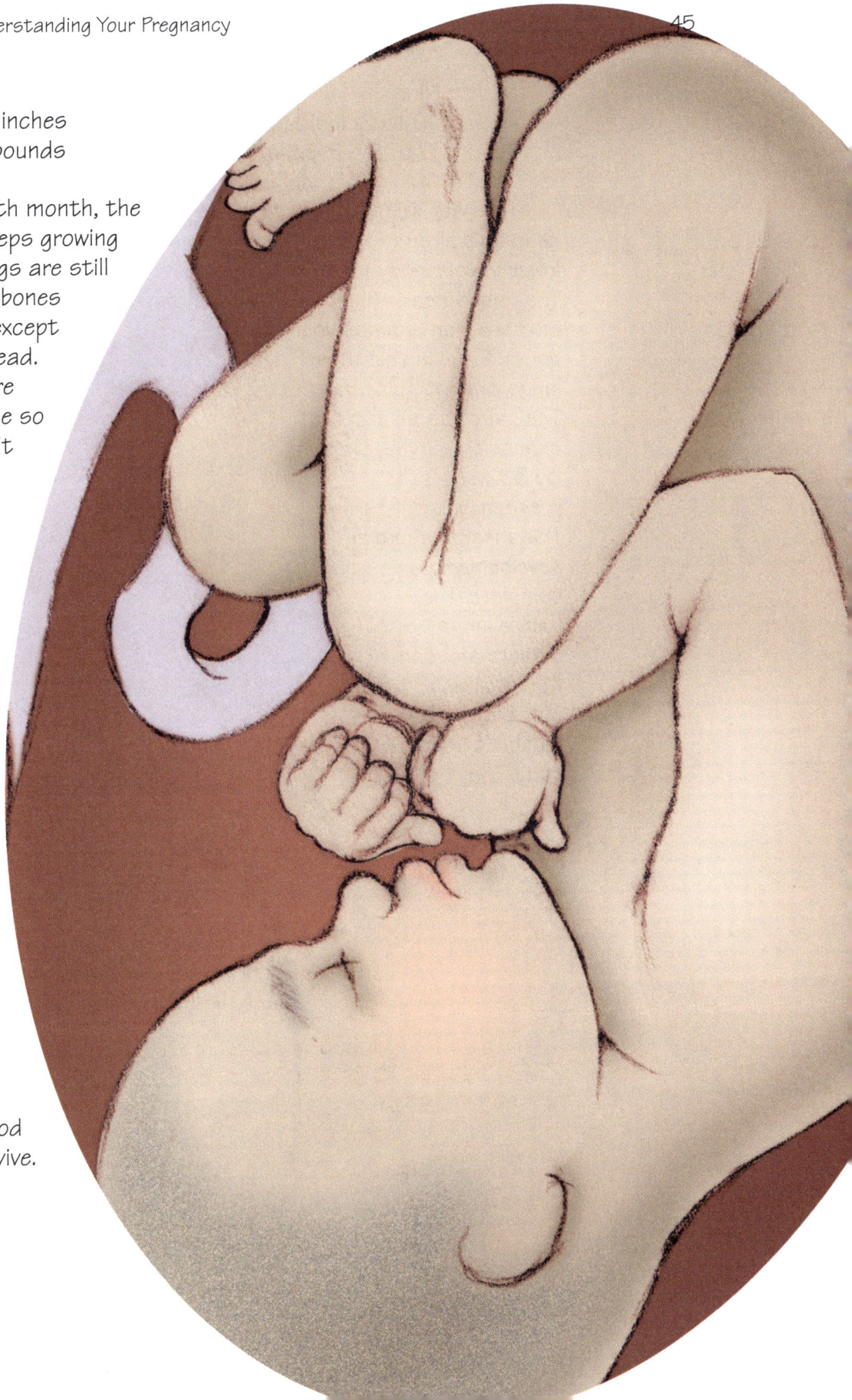

Month Nine
Length: 19 to 21 inches
Weight: 6 to 8½ pounds

The baby will take a head-down position, if he hasn't already. He will "drop" or move lower in your body to prepare for birth. The baby's head will engage (settle into position against your pelvic bone). Early in this month, the lungs are not quite mature. The baby has an excellent chance to survive, though. By 38 weeks, the pregnancy is full-term. This means prenatal development is complete. The baby's lungs are mature and can work well outside the mother's body. The baby is ready to be born.

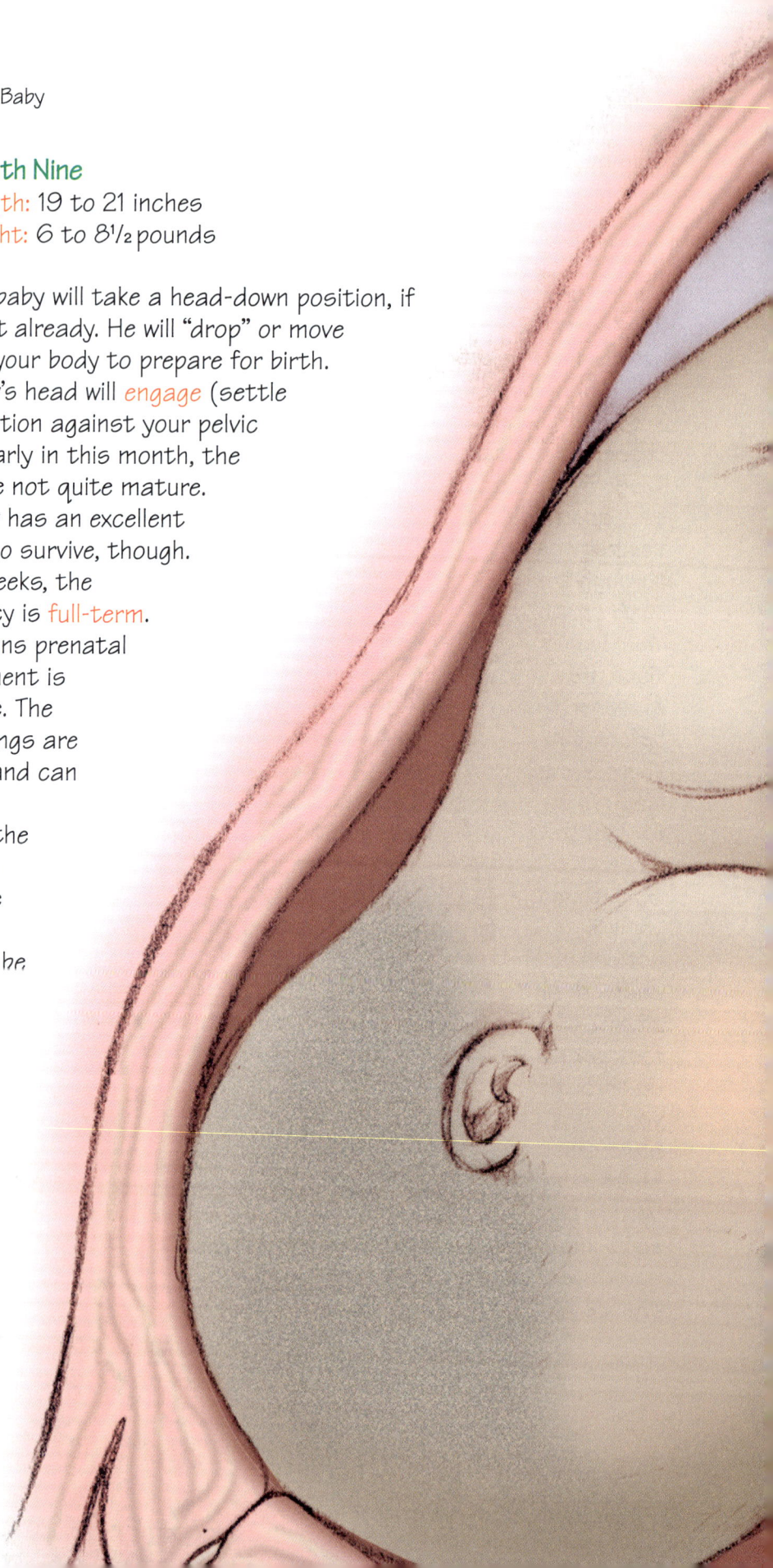

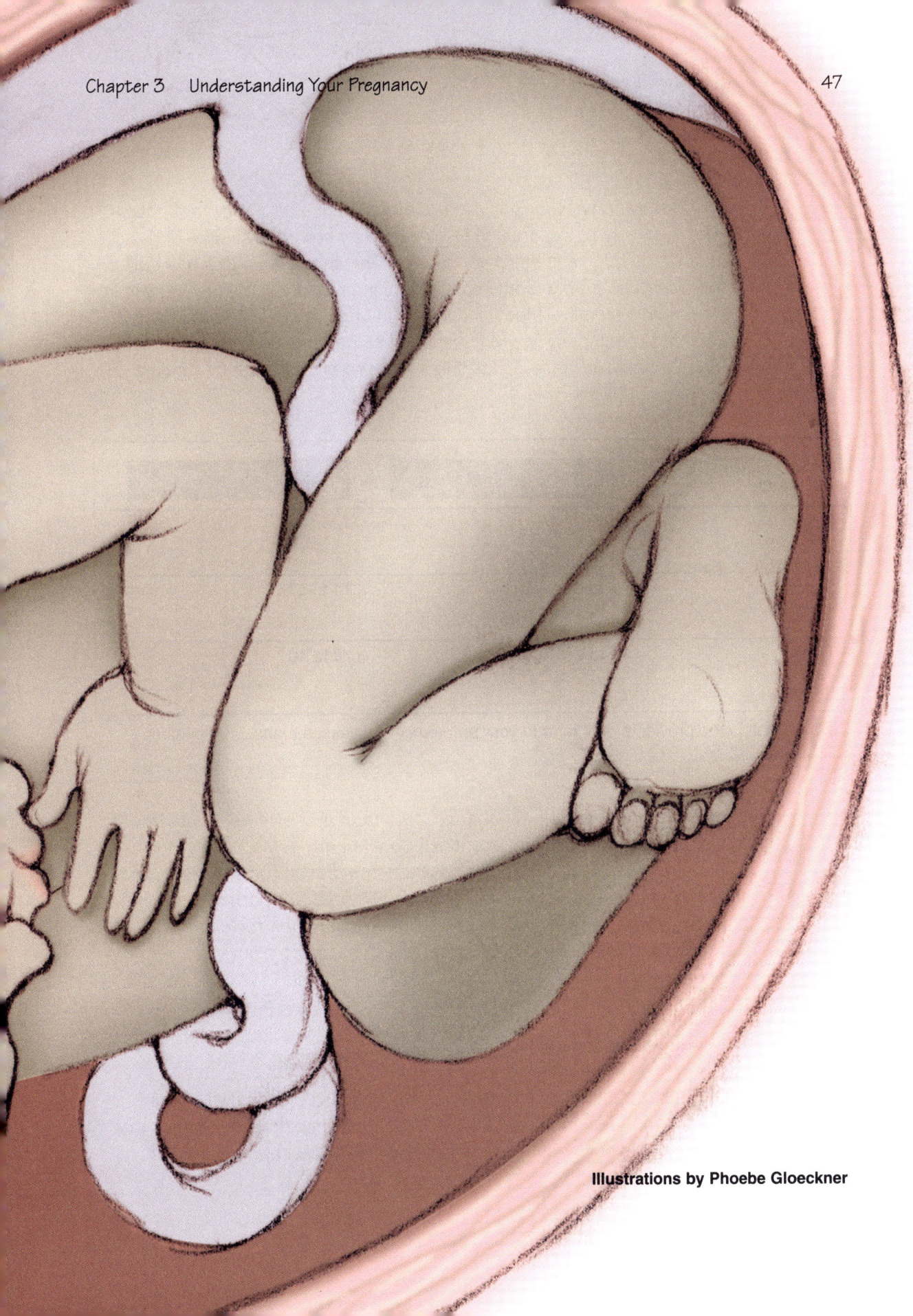

Illustrations by Phoebe Gloeckner

Your Changing Body

Before birth, your baby grows and changes at a very fast rate. The best way to describe this growth is by how many weeks or months it has been since conception. The changes in your body will happen more slowly. Some occur early in pregnancy. Others happen in the middle months. Most occur late in pregnancy. To describe these changes, pregnancy is divided into three parts called trimesters. Each trimester lasts about three months or 13 weeks. See Figure 3-1.

Understanding Trimesters

Trimester	Months	Weeks
First	1 to 3	1 to 13
Second	4 to 6	14 to 27
Third	7 to 9	28 to 40

3-1 Health care providers may refer to your pregnancy in weeks, months, or trimesters.

Your body will slowly change its shape and size as the baby inside you grows. It adjusts itself to the baby's needs. As your pregnancy goes on, you may notice some discomforts. These are a result of the changes within your body. Most are normal. You should know what changes and discomforts are common for each trimester. This will help you know what to expect from your pregnancy. It will also alert you to any problems.

Physical Changes

For the next few months, you will share your body with your baby. It may seem like this tiny person has invaded your space and taken over your body. You may wonder if all the changes in your body are normal. You might think you will never get your body (or your shape) back again. The next sections of this chapter describe these physical changes and give tips for handling them.

Weight Gain

Weight gain is a necessary part of pregnancy. You may wonder why all this weight is needed. You are carrying a baby inside you. This baby and the tissues that support it weigh several pounds. (At birth, most babies weigh between 6 to 8 pounds.) Your body makes more blood during pregnancy to nourish your baby. Your breasts grow to make milk for her. Each of these factors adds to the weight you must gain for a healthy pregnancy. See Figure 3-2.

Weight Gain for Pregnant Teens

Baby	6 to 8½ pounds
Breast increase	1 to 2 pounds
Blood increase	3 to 3½ pounds
Fat	7 to 9 pounds
Body fluid	2 to 3 pounds
Uterus increase	2 to 3 pounds
Placenta	2 to 2½ pounds
Amniotic fluid	2 to 3½ pounds
Total	**25 to 35 pounds**

3-2   During pregnancy, the weight you'll gain goes to the baby, the tissues that support the baby, and the changes in your body created by the pregnancy.

As a teen, you need to gain even more weight during pregnancy than adult women do. This is because your body is trying to complete its own growth. The average recommended weight gain for pregnant teens is 25 to 35 pounds. Your health care provider will tell you what is the right amount for you.

This amount will be based on your age, height, and prepregnancy weight. If you were underweight before pregnancy, you may need to gain closer to 35 pounds. The same is true if you are younger than 15 years of age. If you were overweight before pregnancy, you may be advised to gain less.

If you gain the right amount, you can likely return to your prepregnancy weight within a few months after delivery. If you gain less, your baby's needs and your body's needs will not be met. You will deprive both of you of the nutrients needed to grow. Gaining much more weight than you should is not good either. This could signal a problem. Also, you should not try to lose weight during pregnancy. This can be dangerous for you and your baby.

Your health care provider should monitor your weight gain throughout your pregnancy. Be sure to tell your health care provider if any of the following happen:

- ☛ You gain much more weight than advised.
- ☛ You have trouble gaining weight.
- ☛ You lose weight.

Some pregnant women are very upset about all the weight they gain. They feel they are fat or unattractive. They may be scared about losing weight after the baby is born. If feelings like these bother you, remember <u>why</u> you are gaining this weight. This may help you see things differently.

Breast Changes

Early in pregnancy, your breasts will probably swell some and be sore. They are preparing to make milk to feed the baby. This soreness should last only a few weeks. As your pregnancy progresses, some liquid may leak from your nipples. This is normal. If the liquid has blood in it, tell your health care provider. Otherwise, you can just ignore it. You can wear cotton pads in your bra to catch the liquid if needed.

Stretch Marks

Many pregnant women get stretch marks. These are dark reddish marks that appear on the skin. They are most common on the abdomen, hips, buttocks, and breasts. Stretch marks happen because the tissue beneath the skin tears as the skin stretches. The tendency to get stretch marks is a trait you inherit from your parents. No creams, lotions, or other products have been proven to reduce or get rid of stretch marks. Moisturizing creams and lotions are good for the skin, though. You can use them to reduce the itchiness of the abdomen in later pregnancy when the skin is very stretched.

Skin Darkening

Some areas of the skin may become darker as a result of pregnancy. First, the area around your nipples, called the areola (uh-REE-uh-luh) may turn darker. The thin line from your belly button to your pubic hair may get darker, too. In some women, parts of the facial skin may darken. This is called the mask of pregnancy. These changes are easier to see in darker-skinned people. After pregnancy, these dark areas slowly start to fade.

Varicose Veins

Pregnant women may develop varicose veins. This is a condition in which the blood vessels in the legs are swollen and enlarged. The veins stick out from the skin more than usual. They can be painful and interfere with walking. Hormones make the blood vessels stretch more easily during pregnancy. Extra weight gain and standing in one place for long periods may also lead to varicose veins. The tendency to develop this condition can also be inherited.

To avoid varicose veins, try the following:

- Gain only as much weight as your health care provider recommends for you.
- Put your feet up when you sit.
- Exercise often (if it's okay with your health care provider).
- Move your legs frequently if you must stand in one place more than a few minutes.

Continuing Body Changes

Early in pregnancy, many changes occur as the body adjusts. These changes were described in detail in Chapter 2. A woman might have nausea and vomiting. She might also have increased urination, fatigue, and breast swelling.

The second trimester is often the most comfortable time of pregnancy. At the start of this trimester, your uterus will start to expand into your abdomen. By 20 weeks, a slight bulge will be noticeable starting near your belly button. Around this time you will feel your baby move. At first, it will be just a brief flutter. It might feel like a feather, butterfly, or bubble moving inside you. As the movements get stronger, you will know your baby is flexing her muscles. There is less pressure on your bladder now. You won't have to urinate as often. By the end of this trimester, the baby will be quite active.

During the third trimester, your body curves will be much more noticeable. The uterus will expand as high as your ribs and as low as your pelvis. Your ribs may be a little sore as the uterus crowds them. The uterus also presses against your lungs, stomach, and bladder. You may be short of breath, have indigestion, and need to urinate frequently. As the birth gets closer, you are likely to feel less comfortable. In the last few weeks, you may find it harder to walk and sit. See Figure 3-3 for some tips to use late in pregnancy.

Comfort Tips for Late Pregnancy

Late in pregnancy, you will probably feel uncomfortable more of the time. Your body is consumed by the baby, and it may seem your pregnancy will last forever. Following these tips may help you feel more comfortable until the baby comes:

❖ Eat smaller meals, but eat more often.

❖ Lessen the pressure on your lungs and stomach by sitting up straight. Avoid slouching.

❖ Sleep on your left side with pillows behind your head and back. You may need to prop a few pillows around you to find a comfortable position.

❖ Be careful not to fall. Changes in your body size and shape can interfere with your balance.

❖ Give yourself more time to get places. The changes in your body may slow you down some.

3-3   Toward the end of pregnancy, it's harder to get comfortable. Following these tips can help.

Normal Discomforts

Some discomforts are a normal part of pregnancy. They result from the many changes in your body that support your growing baby. At times, you may feel pretty uncomfortable. It may help if you remember that pregnancy lasts only a few months. Soon you will have your body all to yourself again. For now, you can learn some ways to cope with these annoying problems.

Try not to feel scared about these discomforts. Each woman's body reacts to pregnancy in its own way. If you are like most women, you will have some, but not all, of these discomforts. If you're one of the few women who don't notice any of them, be glad—you're lucky!

Nausea and Vomiting

For many women, nausea and vomiting are the hardest discomforts to handle. The nausea that happens in pregnancy is often called morning sickness. This name isn't accurate—nausea can occur any time of day or night. The effects can vary a great deal. You may just feel waves of mild nausea. Some women lose their appetites. You may be very sensitive to a certain odor. This odor may seem to trigger nausea. You might feel sick to your stomach and vomit from time to time. In severe cases, women have severe nausea and vomiting that lasts for several months.

If nausea and vomiting are a problem, try the following:

- Avoid strong odors when possible. Perfumes, aftershave lotions, cigarette smoke, or cooking odors may be the biggest problems.
- Keep a piece of fresh lemon with you. Many women report a fresh lemon scent helps reduce nausea.
- Tea made with fresh ginger reduces nausea for some.
- Get the equivalent of 8 to 10 glasses of fluid a day. Foods with a high water content, such as watermelon and grapes, may help. High fluid intake may reduce nausea.
- Eat a few crackers before getting out of bed.

☞ If you can't keep solid foods down, try clear liquids such as water, apple juice, and ginger ale. Sometimes ice chips and popsicles will help.

☞ If you can't keep any fluids down for 24 hours, call your health care provider or go to a local emergency room. You may need intravenous (IV) fluids to prevent dehydration. Dehydration would be dangerous for you and your baby.

☞ Avoid taking any medicines for nausea or vomiting unless your health care provider says you should. Ask if there are safe medicines that help reduce nausea and vomiting.

Frequent Urination

In early pregnancy, you will also have to urinate more often. Your growing uterus is pressing against your bladder. The bladder cannot hold as much urine as normal. This means you will need to use the bathroom more often. This may be annoying, but there is little you can do about it. Don't reduce the amount of fluids you drink. You and your baby need about 8 to 10 glasses of fluid a day. Drinking less than this can be harmful. It may cause you to become dehydrated or develop a urinary tract infection (UTI).

Dizziness

Dizziness means feeling lightheaded or faint. You may feel dizzy if you stand quickly after sitting or reclining. In pregnancy, blood more quickly leaves the brain and pools in the legs. This can be one cause of dizziness. Too little iron or glucose (a form of sugar) in your blood can also cause this feeling. If you feel dizzy often, tell your health care provider.

To avoid or relieve dizziness, try the following tips:

☞ Don't skip meals. Never wait more than four hours to eat something.

☞ When you feel dizzy, sit with your head bent toward your knees for a minute or two. Then get up slowly.

☞ Whenever you rise from a sitting or reclining position, do it slowly.

☛ Avoid very hot baths or showers. Extreme heat can expand the blood vessels in your legs. This will reduce blood flow to your head, which may cause dizziness.

Fatigue

When you are pregnant, your body works harder to help your baby grow. As a result, you may feel more tired and sleepy. Try to sleep at least eight hours every night. Taking a nap in the afternoon may also help. Your eating habits are also important. You need the energy and nutrients healthy foods provide. Eat nutritious meals and ask your health care provider whether you need prenatal vitamins.

Constipation

Constipation means being unable to have a bowel movement or having hard stools. This discomfort is common in pregnancy. It is caused by pressure on your intestines by the growing uterus. It also happens because hormonal changes in pregnancy slow down the bowels.

If constipation is a problem, try the following:

☛ Drink plenty of fluids (8 to 10 glasses a day).

☛ Get moderate exercise every day. Go for a walk. Use stairs instead of an elevator when possible.

☛ Include more fiber in your diet. This will help keep your bowel movements regular. Fiber is in whole-grain products, as well as fresh fruits and vegetables.

☛ Avoid straining to have a bowel movement. Straining can give you hemorrhoids (hih-muh-ROYDZ), which are swollen veins in the rectum. These can be painful. Don't take any laxatives. Your health care provider may prescribe a stool softener.

Heartburn

Heartburn is a burning feeling you might get in your chest. The valve that keeps acids in your stomach loosens in pregnancy. Heartburn happens when some of this acid touches the esophagus.

The esophagus (ee-SAH-fuh-guhs) is the tube that leads from the mouth to the stomach. Heartburn has nothing to do with your heart.

If you have heartburn, try the following:

- Eat smaller, more frequent meals.
- Avoid fried or spicy foods.
- Sleep with more than one pillow behind you. When the top part of your body is raised a little, stomach acid can't rise into the esophagus as easily.
- Try drinking some milk or water.
- Do not take over-the-counter medications for heartburn unless your health care provider has told you it's okay to do so.

Backache

Backache is also common during pregnancy. It happens most in the second and third trimesters. Your swelling abdomen may cause you to shift your weight toward the front of your body. See Figure 3-4. This shift will put strain on your back muscles. You may develop an aching back.

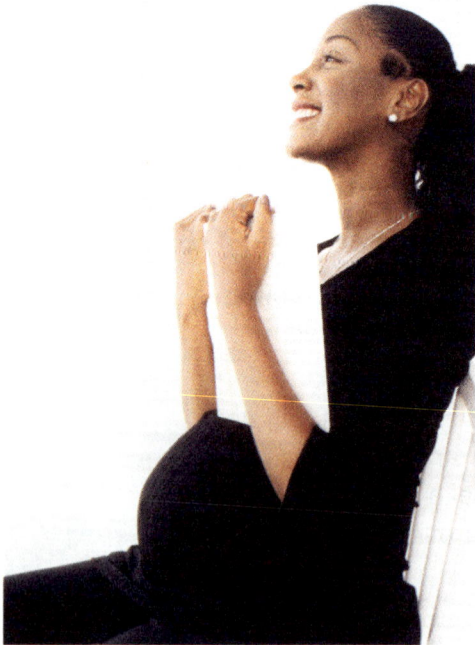

To relieve backaches, try the following:

- When you are standing, tuck your buttocks under a bit. This tends to straighten the curve of your back. Also, bend your knees just a little.
- In a chair, sit with your back against the back of the chair or use a pillow.
- Use a heating pad on your back.
- Take a warm (but not hot) bath.
- Do the pelvic tilt exercise (see Chapter 5).

3-4 As your abdomen grows, it may cause backaches. This is most common near the end of your pregnancy.

Vaginal Changes

You may find you have more discharge from your vagina during pregnancy. This is normal. You can just ignore it unless the discharge itches, burns, or smells bad. These are signs you might have an infection that needs treatment. Don't treat yourself with over-the-counter medicines or creams. Instead, see your health care provider. He or she can examine you to see what is causing the problem. Then your provider can find a safe way to treat the problem.

Your Changing Emotions

Physical changes are not the only changes during pregnancy. You can expect many emotional changes, too. These changes are normal. Many are caused by hormones. Others come from the decisions you must make. These changes are a part of every pregnancy. Each woman handles them in her own way. If you didn't want or expect to be pregnant, you may face extra emotional issues. Be patient with yourself at this time and ask others to be patient with you.

Adjusting to Being Pregnant

In early pregnancy, your body is adjusting to pregnancy. Your mind also has to adjust. At first, you may not believe you are pregnant. Then, you may feel excited about having a baby. At the same time, you may be anxious. You may be afraid of how your family will react. You may worry about how pregnancy will change your life. Relationships with friends, family, and your baby's father may also concern you.

At this time, you may cry more easily. It might take less than usual for you to feel hurt or angry. Some days you may be excited about the pregnancy. Other days you may feel doubtful or anxious. Your moods can change quickly and without warning. You may feel upset for no reason. This can be confusing.

Most pregnant teens find it helpful to talk to someone about how they feel. You may want to talk to a family member. If that's not possible, talk to someone you trust at school. Other people might be a close friend or someone from your house of worship. You and your baby's father also need to talk about what the pregnancy will mean for both of you. This is a good time to begin to plan what the two of you will do since you're pregnant.

Considering Adoption

As you look into your options, you may decide to choose adoption. Your health care provider, social worker, or school nurse can help you contact an adoption agency. These agencies offer counseling. This can help you learn about adoption and decide whether it is right for you. An agency can give you the support you will need to plan an adoption.

Take your time to make this important decision. You want to arrive at the best decision for you and your baby. You'll have to live with whatever choice you make. You don't have to make a final decision until after your baby is born.

If you plan an adoption, you may have mixed feelings. You may wonder how you'll feel afterward. It may feel good to know you're choosing a family for your baby. You may feel sad, too. Most days, you may be sure about the adoption. Other times, you may have doubts. Some people may have a hard time accepting and supporting your decision. Explain to them it is your responsibility to decide whether to plan an adoption for your baby.

Second Trimester Thoughts and Feelings

By the time your second trimester starts, your emotions will likely be more under control. The pregnancy seems more real as the baby begins to move. Your pregnancy will also have begun to show. During these three months, you may think a lot about how the baby will look. You are curious whether the baby will be a boy or a girl. You will think about the kind of mother you want to be. These thoughts and concerns are normal. They are a healthy response to pregnancy. Your family and friends may notice you are less social. You may have to explain this is a normal part of pregnancy.

Young fathers-to-be also experience emotional changes. They wonder what kind of fathers they will be. They think about what they will be able to give their children. A father-to-be may also worry about the health of his partner and the baby. On the other hand, some fathers-to-be may feel upset to have caused pregnancy. They may be in denial. These men may not take responsibility for the baby they've helped create.

Your relationship with the baby's father may become tense at times. This is true whether you're still together or not. It is normal. Talking to one another about your hopes and fears can help. Discussing the decisions you have to make is also good. See Figure 3-5.

Your relationship with the baby's father should not be abusive or controlling. It is not okay for him to abuse you. Physical or emotional abuse could hurt you and your growing baby. Trying to control whom you see or where you go is also abusive. Abuse usually does not stop on its own. It often continues or gets worse during pregnancy.

If your partner is abusing you, your life and your baby's life may be in danger. Tell an adult you trust or your health care provider. You can also call a hotline for victims of abuse. Seek help in ending the relationship and being safe. You and your baby deserve it.

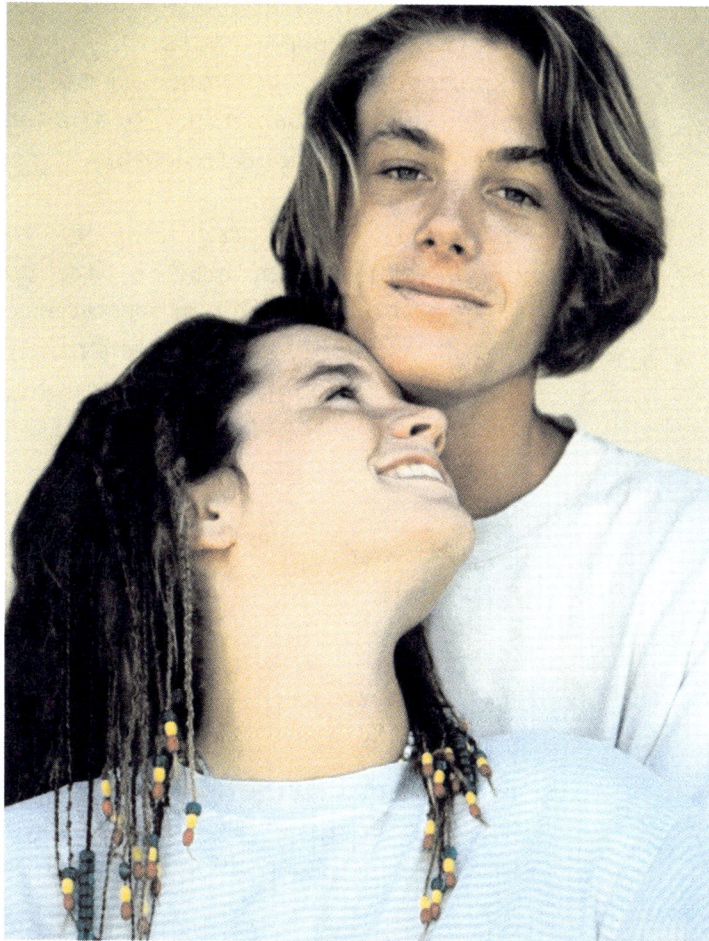

3-5 Having a strong relationship with your baby's father can help you cope with the changes pregnancy brings.

Third Trimester Thoughts and Feelings

During the last three months of pregnancy, you may find some anxiety returns. You may start to wonder how you will feel during the birth. You're glad to be close to the end of pregnancy. On the other hand, you may be scared about labor and delivery. All women worry about the safety of their babies and themselves. Many women have strange or frightening dreams during this time. These dreams are common. They do not mean anything is wrong with you or your baby.

During this time, it is also normal to turn your thoughts inward. You may spend a lot of time thinking about things. Hurtful past experiences may come to mind. If past experiences trouble you, talk to someone about it. A counselor, trusted adult, or friend can listen and help you work through these feelings.

At the end of pregnancy, you may be pretty uncomfortable. You may be tired but unable to sleep. You may feel nervous, grouchy, or irritable. Try to relax as much as possible. Soon your pregnancy will be over. Your baby will be born. That thought will help you bear the discomfort you feel. Pregnancy is only temporary—it won't last forever.

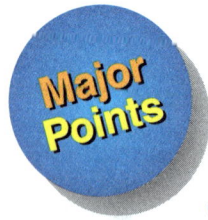

Major Points

☛ Chromosomes are the parts of cells that carry the traits we inherit from our parents. One set of chromosomes decides whether a baby will be a boy or girl.

☛ The baby grows and changes rapidly over the 40 weeks of pregnancy. Its support system includes the placenta, umbilical cord, amniotic sac, and amniotic fluid.

☛ Pregnancy can be divided into three parts called trimesters. Each trimester brings physical changes in your body. The third trimester will be the most uncomfortable part for you.

☛   Weight gain is necessary to provide what your body needs to help the baby to grow. Ask your health care provider how much weight to gain and how to gain the right amount.

☛   Some discomforts of pregnancy are normal. Try to find ways to deal with these discomforts and remember they are temporary.

☛   Emotional changes are common throughout pregnancy. Hormones influence your moods. The changes that pregnancy (and the coming baby) brings to your life do, too.

Chapter 4
Having a Healthy
Pregnancy

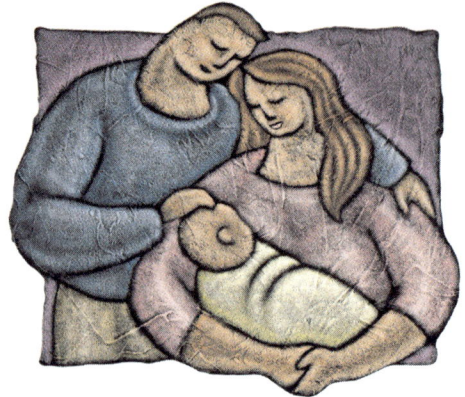

Whether you will be parenting your baby or making an adoption plan, you will want to give your child the best possible start. You can do much to keep yourself and your baby healthy. Practicing good health habits is the first step. Seeking medical care is also important. Babies are healthiest when their mothers are healthy. Your baby's health depends on you.

Every pregnancy has risks, but the younger you are, the greater the risk is. Just being a teen puts your pregnancy at a higher risk. Pregnant teens who are 15 years old or younger have the most problems. Their babies are the most likely to be born too small, too early, or both. These babies also have more health problems after birth.

Good health is even more important for pregnant teens. Teens have more problems in pregnancy. One reason relates directly to age. A teen mother's body is still growing at a fast pace. Her nutrient needs are high. Her body may not be ready to support a growing baby. The baby gets all the nutrients and oxygen it needs from its mother's body. A teen's body may not yet have stored enough nutrients to meet her own needs in addition to her baby's. That is why younger teens are advised to gain more weight and consume more calories during pregnancy.

This chapter will explain how you can stay healthy during pregnancy. You will learn about the importance of medical care. This chapter also explains how unhealthy behaviors can harm your baby.

Medical Care During Pregnancy

Lack of early medical care puts pregnant teens at high risk. As a group, teens are less likely than other women to seek care early in pregnancy. Studies show one in three pregnant teens lack medical care in the first trimester.

A teen should seek medical care as soon as she suspects she is pregnant. This will greatly lower the risks she and her baby face. Medical care given in pregnancy is called prenatal care. If you have not already begun prenatal care, do so right away. Be sure to keep all your appointments. This way your health care provider can make sure your pregnancy is going as it should. Do all you can to keep you and your baby healthy. Prenatal care is a good start.

Providers of Prenatal Care

You can get prenatal care in a doctor's office, hospital, clinic, or community health center. Some school-based health clinics also give prenatal care. If you don't know where to go, look in the phone book under Pregnancy.

You may wonder who can provide prenatal care. A few types of health care providers can do this. An obstetrician (ahb-STUH-trish-un) is a doctor whose specialty is prenatal care and childbirth. See Figure 4-1. A family practice doctor treats all kinds of patients. He or she has had enough training to provide prenatal care and deliver babies.

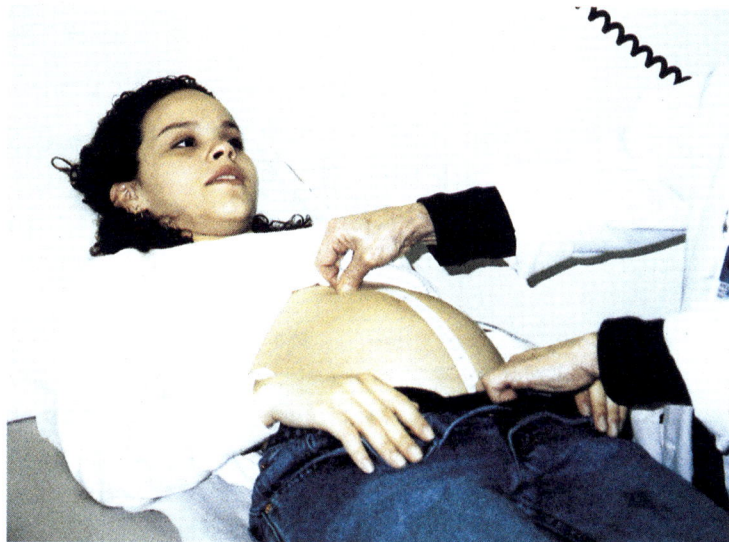

4-1 This obstetrician has been specially trained to provide care for pregnant women. She is measuring the size of the uterus to see how much the baby has grown.

Some nurses can provide care for pregnant women. A certified nurse-midwife is trained to give prenatal care and deliver babies. A nurse practitioner (NP) has special education and training in women's health. An NP can give prenatal care but cannot deliver babies. A doctor or certified nurse-midwife would have to do this.

Think of your health care provider as part of your team. This team includes all the people working to bring your baby into the world! The team's goal is for your baby to be born safely and for both of you to be healthy. Work with your health care provider to make this happen.

First Prenatal Visit

You may have already had your first prenatal visit. If not, you should go soon. If you're like other teens, you may want to know what to expect. This first visit will likely last longer than later visits. Your blood pressure and weight will be checked. It will also include the following:

- a medical history
- a physical examination, including a pelvic exam
- calculation of your due date
- some blood tests and/or prenatal tests
- advice on nutrition, exercise, and lifestyle habits during pregnancy

Medical History

Your health care provider will ask about your medical history. See Figure 4-2. You will pass some health traits to your child. Knowing your history will alert your provider to any problems that may affect your pregnancy. Your parents will know your family's health history. If you can, talk to your baby's father and his family. Find out about their health history. The baby will inherit health traits from them, too.

You will be asked about any past pregnancies or STIs. Your provider will want to know if you use alcohol, tobacco, or drugs. It can be hard to answer such personal questions. Be honest, though.

What Does My Medical History Include?

❖ Hospitalization record—a list of each date you were hospitalized and the condition for which you were hospitalized (mother-to-be and father-to-be).

❖ Serious illness record—a list of major illnesses you have or have had (mother-to-be, father-to-be, and their families).

❖ Inherited disorders or disabilities that run in the family (families of mother-to-be and father-to-be).

❖ Allergies (mother-to-be).

❖ Record of previous pregnancies (mother-to-be).

❖ Knowledge of current STIs (mother-to-be and father-to-be). History of past STIs (mother-to-be).

❖ History of alcohol, tobacco, and other drug use (mother-to-be).

❖ Other factors as determined by the health care provider.

4-2 A complete medical history can alert your health care provider to possible problems with you or the baby.

Your answers allow your provider to give you the best possible care. He or she won't tell anyone what you've shared. If you have special concerns about privacy, talk to your provider without anyone else in the room.

Pelvic Exam

A complete physical exam will be done. It will include a two-part pelvic exam. The first part is done with a speculum. This instrument is gently inserted into the vagina. The walls of the vagina are very elastic. The speculum holds these muscles open. This lets your health care provider see your vagina and cervix.

With the speculum in place, it is easy to test for some STIs. These tests are done to be sure your baby is protected from getting these diseases. Others require blood tests, which can also be done at this visit.

The speculum is also needed to do a Pap test. This test can show abnormal cells that could develop into cervical cancer. To do this test, your provider will use a special small plastic or wooden stick. A Pap test is done by gently brushing some cells from the cervix. These cells are then sent to a laboratory. Here, they are examined under a microscope.

The second part of the pelvic exam is the bimanual. Your health care provider will insert two fingers into your vagina. He or she will place the other hand on your abdomen. By doing this, your provider can estimate the size of your uterus. This tells him or her how far along your pregnancy is. In the bimanual exam, the provider can also examine your pelvic bones. This is a check to see if there is enough room for the baby to pass through during birth.

The pelvic exam will only last a few minutes. It will be easier if you can relax. Taking a few deep breaths might help. If it is your first pelvic exam or you feel anxious, tell your health care provider. You might find it comforting to have someone you trust with you during the exam. Afterward, most teens say the pelvic exam is not as bad as they thought it would be.

Estimating Your Due Date

One of your big questions may be when your baby will be born. At this first visit, your health care provider will give you a due date. This date tells when you can expect your baby to be born. To get this date, your provider will ask you when the first day of your last normal menstrual period was. Your baby should be born about 40 weeks from this date. An easy formula can be used to find the due date. See Figure 4-3.

When Is My Baby Due?

1. First, write down in numbers the date your last normal menstrual period started. *April 14 or 4/14.*

2. Add seven to the day number. *14+7=21. 4/21 or April 21.*

3. Subtract three from the month number. *4-3=1. 1/21 or next January 21.*

If your last period started April 14, your baby will be due next January 21.

4-3   Use this simple calculation to estimate your baby's due date.

Your due date is only an estimate. Most babies are born within about two weeks of this date. The due date will be less accurate if your menstrual cycle hasn't been regular. If you know the date of conception, you may think the due date doesn't seem right. Health care providers count the weeks starting with the first day of the last menstrual period. Usually, conception occurs about two weeks after this. If your baby was conceived about three weeks ago, your provider would likely say you're about five weeks pregnant.

Prenatal Tests

Your first visit may include a few prenatal tests. Your blood will be tested for its type and iron content. A urine test will check for protein and sugar. (High levels can signal problems.) Tests can be done for STIs, as well as other infections and illnesses.

You may want to be tested for HIV (human immunodeficiency virus) at this time. HIV testing has become one of the routine prenatal blood tests. This test tells whether you have the virus that causes a life-threatening illness called AIDS (acquired immunodeficiency syndrome). This virus has no cure, but you need to know whether you have it. If you do, your health care provider can give you special medicines. These will lower the risk that your baby will get the virus. If you have HIV, starting these medicines early may even save your baby's life. (You can learn more about HIV and AIDS in another title in this series, Understanding Your Changing Life.)

Your prenatal blood test may also include a test for cystic fibrosis (CF) to see if you carry a trait for CF. CF is a serious lung disease that your baby might have if both you and your baby's father have the trait. You may also be tested for the sickle cell trait, which can cause an inherited blood disease.

At the first visit, an ultrasound test may be recommended. The ultrasound test uses sound waves to make a video "picture" of the baby. This picture is called a sonogram. Ultrasound is not needed or done in every pregnancy. It can show certain problems with the baby and can confirm the age of the fetus. To do an ultrasound, a small sensor is placed on your abdomen or in your vagina. You can see the baby on a screen like that of a TV. You may also be able to get a copy of the sonogram pictures.

Later Prenatal Visits

Pregnant teens need more frequent prenatal care than adult women. Teens have a greater risk of developing problems in pregnancy. See Figure 4-4. Seeing your health care provider more often can help you avoid these problems. Your provider will tell you how often to schedule prenatal visits. After the first prenatal visit, your visits will be shorter. A routine visit usually consists of the following:

- ☞ blood pressure check
- ☞ urine test for sugar and protein
- ☞ weight check
- ☞ measure of the fundal height (distance from the pelvis to the top of the uterus) to see how much the baby has grown
- ☞ listening to the fetal heartbeat (after 12 weeks)
- ☞ checking the baby's movement (after 20 weeks)

Prenatal Tests

At your later prenatal visits, more tests may be done if there is a specific concern. Even if your health care provider suggests these tests, it is your decision. Ask questions. Find out why a test

Warning Signs

Call your health care provider if you have any of the following:
- ❖ vaginal bleeding
- ❖ persistent pain or cramping
- ❖ headache that doesn't go away
- ❖ swelling, especially of the hands, face, and feet
- ❖ pain when you urinate
- ❖ vaginal itching
- ❖ fluid leaking from your vagina

4-4 You should also contact your health care provider if you notice any of these warning signs.

is needed and what the risks are. If you need help deciding, you may want to ask your parents for their input. You can also seek a second opinion from another health care provider.

Ultrasound can be done at the first prenatal visit. It may also be needed at any time after that. Ultrasound is used mainly when there are concerns about the baby's health or to determine the due date. If done after the fourth month, ultrasound may be able to reveal a baby's gender.

During your fourth month, you may be offered a blood test called a maternal serum alpha-fetoprotein (muh-TUHR-nuhl SIH-ruhm AL-fuh-fee-toh-PROH-teen) test. This test, often called the MSAFP, screens for Down syndrome as well as specific problems with the baby's brain and spinal cord. An abnormal result means further tests are needed. It doesn't mean there is a definite problem with the baby. Additional tests may show there isn't a problem.

In amniocentesis (am-NEE-oh-sen-TEE-suhs), a little amniotic fluid is taken from the uterus with a needle. This needle is inserted through the abdomen. The fluid is then tested to reveal certain physical problems with the baby. An ultrasound is done along with this test so the health care provider can see the baby on the screen. This way the provider won't harm the baby while doing the test.

Amniocentesis is not often done in teen pregnancies. Your provider may recommend it if he or she thinks your baby might have a certain inherited disorder. This test is usually done in the fourth month. There is a slight risk of miscarriage after an amniocentesis.

Pregnancy Complications

Most pregnancies progress with few or no problems. Others have more trouble. A number of complications can occur during pregnancy. If you know what they are, you can recognize the symptoms if they occur.

Regular prenatal checkups can find some of these problems early so they don't become serious. Healthful lifestyle choices can also prevent many of them. In some cases it isn't clear why a complication occurs.

Premature Labor

Premature labor is labor that begins before week 37 of pregnancy. If this labor is not stopped, it will result in a premature birth. A premature baby may not be developed enough to survive. He may not be able to develop normally outside the mother's body. Often, his lungs cannot supply enough oxygen to his body. Bleeding can develop in the brain.

Very premature babies (those born at six or seven months) have many more complications than those born later. With each week the pregnancy continues, the baby gets closer to finishing his development.

Premature labor can occur for a few different reasons. Using tobacco, drugs, or alcohol during pregnancy can increase the risk. Some infections can also cause premature labor.

If labor starts too early, it can sometimes be delayed until the baby matures a little more. The proper medications and bed rest may be able to stop the contractions. These treatments must be started as soon as possible, though. Waiting can cause the labor to continue to the point where it cannot be stopped. For this reason, if you have any of the following signs, call your health care provider at once:

Uterine Contractions. If you have more than four contractions in one hour, this is a warning sign. Contractions may feel like the cramps you get with your period. During a contraction, your abdomen will get hard. It will soften again as the contraction goes away. When contractions begin, they may not be painful.

Pelvic Pressure. Sometimes a contraction will start as a feeling of pressure in your lower abdomen or vagina. This pressure lasts no matter how you move. It is often created by the baby's head pressing against the pelvic bone.

Change in Vaginal Discharge. The amount or kind of vaginal discharge may suddenly change. You might have more discharge. It may be thick and sticky or watery with some blood in it. Note these changes so you can tell your health care provider.

Low Backache. You may have an ache in your lower back that comes and goes or is constant. A constant backache may signal the beginning of labor. Aches that come and go may actually be early contractions.

Low Birthweight

A low-birthweight baby is one who weighs less than 5½ pounds at birth. Low-birthweight babies have a much greater chance of health problems at birth and later in life. When they are born, their lungs and brains are not fully developed. These small babies get sick more easily and are hospitalized more often. See Figure 4-5.

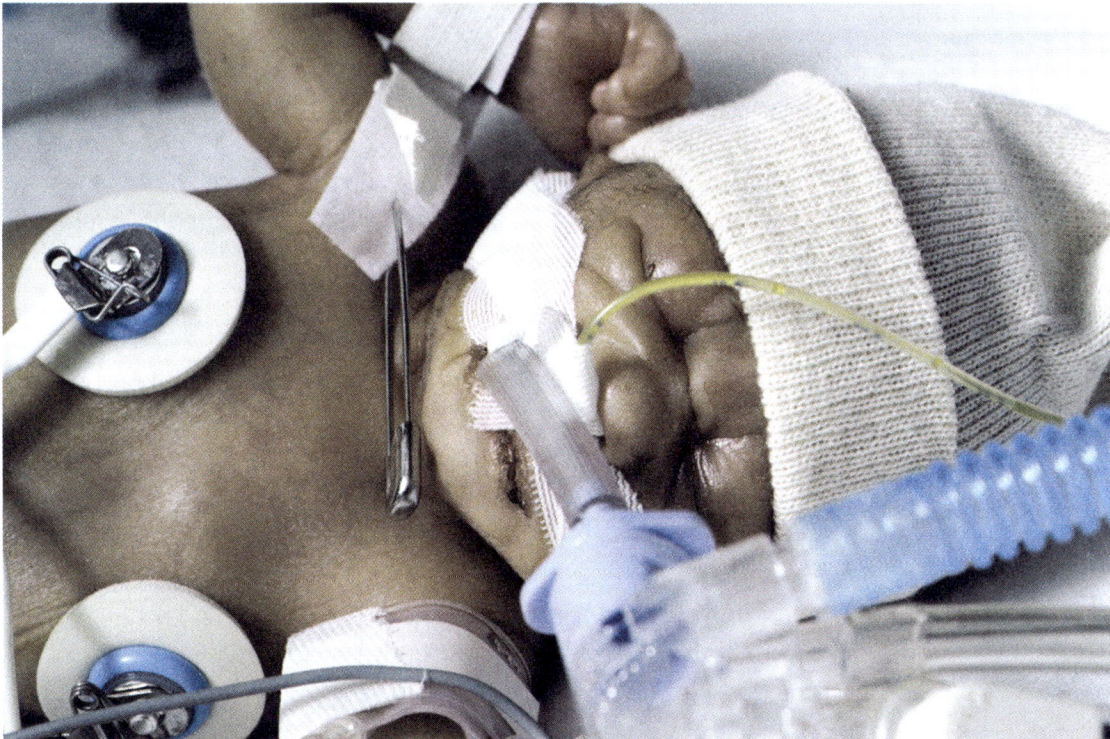

4-5 This premature, low-birthweight baby is seriously ill. She must stay in the hospital quite a while. Various tubes and monitors attached to the baby help the doctors take care of her.

72   Your New Baby

Some of the effects don't show right away. Low birthweight has been linked to problems with development, health, and behavior. As they get older, low-birthweight infants may also have learning disabilities.

Teens are at high risk for having low-birthweight babies. The following factors raise your chance of having a low-birthweight baby:

- not getting early, regular prenatal care
- not gaining the right amount of weight during pregnancy
- not eating enough healthful foods
- using drugs, alcohol, or tobacco

These factors are under your control. Make healthful choices in these areas while you're pregnant. This is the best way to help your baby gain enough weight before birth. Having an average birthweight will give her a much healthier start.

Anemia

Anemia (uh-NEE-mee-uh) is a condition caused by not enough iron in the blood. Iron is an essential nutrient—you need a certain amount of it every day. Iron plays a major role in the body. It does the following:

- builds red blood cells
- assists red blood cells in carrying oxygen through the body
- releases some of the energy in other nutrients
- helps you feel energized
- makes antibodies to fight infection

You need more iron during pregnancy. The placenta that supports your baby is growing. It is rich with blood vessels and tissue. Your body is making more blood to support the pregnancy. It also helps your baby's body make his own blood supply. Your baby also takes iron from your body to build his own iron stores. He will need these stores to provide his body with iron for his first few months of life. Each of these tasks requires extra iron over your body's normal needs.

Many teens are anemic before pregnancy. Their diets have not been healthful. In pregnancy, this anemia tends to get worse. Other teens were not anemic before pregnancy but couldn't meet the increased demands of pregnancy. No matter how it develops, anemia can cause health problems for mother and baby. See Figure 4-6.

You might wonder if you have anemia. Signs of anemia include the following:

- getting tired easily (beyond normal pregnancy fatigue)
- feeling short of breath
- feeling lightheaded or dizzy often
- having a pale appearance

Eating nutritious foods can give you the iron you need. Be sure to take any iron tablets your health care provider prescribes for you. If you are concerned about anemia, talk to your provider. He or she knows how much you need and how you can get it.

Pregnancy-Induced Hypertension

High blood pressure that develops in pregnancy or right after the baby is born is called pregnancy-induced hypertension (PIH). You might also hear this condition called preeclampsia (pre-ih-KLAMP-see-uh), toxemia (tahk-SEE-mee-uh), or PET. Its cause is unknown. If a woman has PIH, her blood pressure begins to increase. She may have a lot of swelling and too much protein in her urine.

Risks of Anemia in Pregnancy

- premature birth
- low-birthweight baby
- severe bleeding after delivery
- mother may feel tired, depressed, irritable, and less healthy
- anemia in the baby

4-6 During pregnancy, anemia can be dangerous to both mother and baby.

If PIH is treated early, both mother and baby can avoid serious health problems. This is why your blood pressure is checked at each prenatal visit. Protein levels are checked in each urine sample you give.

If they aren't treated early, the effects of PIH can be severe. High blood pressure could damage your eyes, kidneys, brain, and liver. Untreated PIH may even result in seizures and death of the mother. It will also reduce the flow of oxygen and nutrients to your baby. This interferes with her growth, causes mental disabilities, and can lead to death.

PIH occurs often in pregnant teens. The following signs may mean you are developing PIH:

- an unexplained weight gain of more than two pounds per week
- swelling of the face, hands, and feet
- persistent headache
- visual changes, especially seeing flashes of light
- persistent upper abdominal pain

Contact your health care provider at once if you have any of these signs. If you have PIH, your provider can help you manage this condition. This will help you and your baby avoid serious problems.

Infections

Some types of infection can seriously harm you or your baby in pregnancy or at birth. Examples are chicken pox, group B strep, tuberculosis (tu-buhr-kyuh-LOH-suhs), rubella (roo-BEH-luh), and toxoplasmosis (tahk-so-plaz-MOH-suhs). Each poses a serious risk in pregnancy. See Figure 4-7. Do all you can to avoid exposure to these infections. Limit contact with people who have them. If you think you may have been exposed to an infection, call your health care provider at once.

Sexually Transmitted Infections

Sexually transmitted infections (STIs) are those that are spread from one person to another during sexual activity. These infections are also called sexually transmitted diseases (STDs).

Infections That Can Complicate Pregnancy

Infection	Description	How It's Spread	What It Can Do	Prevention/ Treatment
Chicken pox (Varicella)	Itchy rash that may spread over entire body. Small, pink spots that turn into blisters and then form scabs. Mild fever.	It's very contagious! You can catch it by being near someone who has it. It becomes contagious two days before the rash appears.	Baby can develop physical or mental disabilities or chicken pox. In third trimester, mother can develop serious pneumonia, which may cause death.	If you've had it, you probably won't get it again. Avoid contact with anyone with a rash. Medicine given within four days of exposure can lower the risk of infection.
Group B Strep	An infection caused by a common bacterium.	Commonly found on the body. Can be passed to newborn during delivery.	Can cause a very serious infection in the newborn. Can infect the mother's uterus at delivery.	Can test for it in last trimester of pregnancy. Can treat during labor with antibiotics.
Tuberculosis	Dangerous lung infection. Can cause serious illness and death. Has no symptoms in its early stages.	It's contagious. You can catch it by being near some-one who has it.	During pregnancy, the disease may become more serious. The baby can contract this disease from the mother after birth.	Avoid contact with infected persons. A test can detect exposure to the germ. A chest X ray confirms the infection. After birth, medicine can be given to prevent the infection.
Rubella (German measles)	Rash that usually starts in the face and neck, swollen lymph glands, and fever.	It's contagious. Spread by direct contact with items contaminated by germs from an infected person.	May cause miscar-riage or stillbirth. Can cause serious vision, hearing, or heart disabilities in the baby.	Can prevent it with a vaccine given *before* or after (not during) pregnancy. Avoid contact with infected persons.
Toxoplasmosis	An infection that is caused by a parasite. Usually has no symptoms. Sometimes fever, sore throat, rash, and swollen glands develop.	You can get it by eating raw or undercooked meat, digging in the garden without gloves, or emptying a cat's litter box.	May cause serious illness in the baby or affect the baby's growth. Can cause miscarriage or premature birth.	Can be prevented by eating well-cooked meat, using gloves in the garden, and not emptying the litter box. There is no effective treatment.

4-7 Keeping yourself free from infections can help you have a healthy pregnancy.

Antibiotics can cure some STIs. Others have no known cure. Some infect the baby in pregnancy, while others pass to him during delivery. See Figure 4-8 for a chart that shows the possible effects of STIs on you and your baby.

How Can STIs Complicate My Pregnancy?

Sexually Transmitted Infection	Effects on Mother and Baby	Treatment/Care
HIV	Can infect the baby during pregnancy, delivery, or breast-feeding. Causes AIDS, a life-threatening illness that can't be cured. Mother's HIV infection can get worse during pregnancy.	Medicine given to the mother during pregnancy can greatly reduce the chance the baby will get the virus. It can also prevent her infection from getting worse. After birth, the baby will need to take medicine, too. No cure.
Chlamydia	Can cause serious eye and lung infections in a baby exposed at birth. May cause premature birth or miscarriage.	Can cure the mother with antibiotics before the baby is born Can treat newborn's eyes with an antibiotic to prevent infection.
Gonorrhea	Can cause stillbirth or premature delivery. Can affect baby's growth. Can infect the baby's eyes at birth, and may cause blindness.	Can cure the mother with antibiotics before the baby is born. Can treat baby's eyes at birth to prevent infection.
Herpes	Can infect the baby during delivery. Can cause miscarriage or stillbirth; disabilities, damage to the baby's eyes and brain, and very serious illness in the baby. May lead to infant death.	May be given a medicine during the ninth month of pregnancy to lower the risk of passing the virus to the baby during birth. Cesarean delivery may be recommended so the baby doesn't pass through the infected birth canal. No cure.
Genital Warts (Human Papilloma Virus)	Can grow large enough to block the birth canal. May cause cervical cancer in the mother. Can cause small growths on the baby's vocal cords.	Medication can sometimes be applied to the warts to keep them small or make them go away. The virus that causes the warts stays in the body, though. No cure, however, a healthy immune system may rid the body of the virus after a few years.

(Continued)

4-8 Sexually transmitted infections can have lasting effects on both mother and child.

How Can STIs Complicate My Pregnancy?

Sexually Transmitted Infection	Effects on Mother and Baby	Treatment/Care
Cytomegalovirus	Can infect the baby during pregnancy. Mother usually has no symptoms. Baby may be born with liver, blood, eye, ear, and brain damage. Mental disabilities and developmental delays may occur.	There is no treatment or cure.
Hepatitis B	Newborn can easily be infected during and shortly after birth. It can damage the liver severely enough to cause death.	Infants can be treated with medicine to prevent the infection. There is no cure once you have the infection. The infection can be prevented with Hepatitis B vaccine.
Syphilis	Can infect the baby during pregnancy. Can cause stillbirth; premature birth; anemia; sores on hands and feet; enlarged liver, spleen, and lymph nodes; and damaged bones, teeth, and kidneys.	Antibiotics given during pregnancy can cure the infection. Antibiotics can be given to the newborn to cure the infection.
Trichomoniasis	Has been associated with premature labor and low birthweight in the infant.	Can take medicine during pregnancy to cure the infection.

4-8 (Continued)

Some STIs can be treated. If an STI can't be cured, your health care provider can still suggest the best possible care to protect the baby. STI tests are done at your first prenatal visit. These can be repeated during your eighth month of pregnancy.

Many times an STI will have no symptoms. If symptoms are present, they may include the following:

- abnormal vaginal discharge
- blister, sore, or bump in the genital area
- abnormal vaginal bleeding or spotting
- abdominal or pelvic pain

During pregnancy, it is easier for infections to enter your body. For this reason, your chance of getting an STI is higher. This risk increases if you have sex with more than one partner. It is also higher if your partner has sex with anyone else. To be safe, you might decide not to have sex while you're pregnant. If you do have sex, using condoms is the only protection for you and your baby against STIs. (For more information about STIs, including symptoms for males, see another title in this series, <u>Understanding Your Changing Life</u>.)

Bacterial Vaginosis

Bacterial vaginosis is a condition associated with sexual intercourse. However, it is not contracted from a partner. It has been associated with premature birth and infection inside the uterus and amniotic sac. The mother can be treated with medication to cure the infection, but it can recur.

Rh Factor

The Rh factor is a substance found in the blood. It has no known function. Most women (about 85 percent) have it. Their blood is called Rh positive (Rh+). If you don't have this factor, your blood is Rh negative (Rh-).

If an Rh- woman is pregnant with an Rh+ baby, it can cause a problem. The blood of the mother and baby are in close contact in the placenta. The mother's blood can detect the Rh factor in the baby's blood. Her body will treat the Rh factor the same way it treats any other unknown substance. It will make antibodies to destroy it. These antibodies can harm or kill the baby. It takes time for the antibodies to build up. They usually do not cause a problem in a woman's first pregnancy. In her next pregnancy, however, the level of antibodies can rise high enough to cause health problems in her second baby.

If you are Rh-, you can receive a shot to prevent your body from making these antibodies. You would have this shot in your seventh month of pregnancy. It is also used right after delivery. If bleeding occurs during pregnancy, the shot can be given then, too.

Gestational Diabetes

Diabetes is an illness in which your body can't use glucose (a type of sugar) in the right way. Gestational (jeh-STAY-shun-uhl) diabetes occurs only in pregnancy. If your blood glucose level is too high, it can harm you and your baby. Diabetic mothers have stillbirths, premature babies, and babies with heart problems more often than other women.

Your health care provider may test you for gestational diabetes between 24 and 28 weeks into the pregnancy. You will drink a special sugary drink. One hour later, you will have blood drawn. If your blood glucose level is too high, you may have gestational diabetes.

Most teens don't develop this illness. If you do, your health care provider can teach you how to control it. You may need insulin shots and strict diet control. Gestational diabetes goes away after pregnancy. It is a sign, however, that you may develop diabetes later.

Gestational diabetes is just one of the many complications that can occur in pregnancy. Don't worry about everything that can go wrong. Many women don't have any of these problems, but it's good to know what can happen. This way you can watch for any signs and report them to your health care provider if they occur.

Reducing the Risks to Mother and Baby

Alcohol, tobacco, and drugs are dangerous to your health. They can be deadly for your unborn baby. If you use these substances in pregnancy, your baby is more likely to die before birth. If she does survive, she will face more health problems than other babies. The harmful effects may not show up for years, but can last a lifetime. Reducing risks keeps you and your baby healthier. See Figure 4-9.

If you're using any of these substances, stop at once! The sooner you stop, the healthier your baby will be. You will have a lower chance of miscarriage, stillbirth, or premature delivery. Some teens find the strength to quit "cold turkey" for the sake of their babies. Thinking of your baby's health may be just the motivation you need.

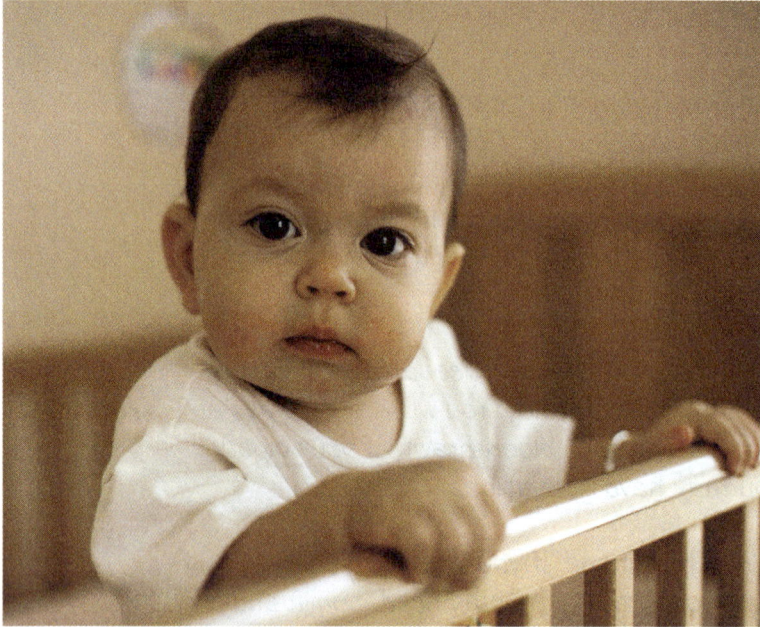

4-9 Taking good care of yourself during pregnancy can help you have a healthy, happy baby.

Others quit a little more gradually by cutting down first. You may find it hard to stop using these substances. If so, talk to your health care provider. He or she can refer you to a counselor or agency that can help.

Avoiding these substances can have another benefit—you can stay out of trouble. Alcohol use is against the law for people under 21 in most states. Tobacco use is illegal for persons younger than 18 in many states. You can be arrested for using illegal substances. You can also be fined, given probation, or sent to a detention center.

Alcohol

Alcohol can damage your unborn baby. It can quickly cross the placenta and enter his blood. The effects could be quite severe. Alcohol stays in a baby's blood longer than in an adult's. Pregnant women who drink alcohol have more low-birthweight babies. They are more likely to miscarry, have a stillbirth, or lose their babies to early infant death.

Alcohol use in pregnancy can also lead to fetal alcohol syndrome (FAS). This condition occurs in the babies of pregnant women who drink heavily. The effects last a lifetime. FAS can cause the following problems:

- physical and mental disabilities
- smaller head and misformed facial features
- very slow rate of growth and development

- ☛ vision and hearing problems
- ☛ behavior and learning problems
- ☛ poor coordination
- ☛ short attention span

The more alcohol you drink, the more severe the effects will be. Even small amounts of alcohol can cause problems, though. There is no known amount of alcohol that is safe during pregnancy. For this reason, the U.S. Surgeon General advises against alcohol use in pregnancy. Alcohol cannot help your baby in any way. It can only cause harm. <u>To protect your baby, do not drink alcohol while you're pregnant!</u>

Tobacco

Tobacco use has been proven to be harmful. It hurts the person smoking and others breathing the smoke. The effects on an unborn baby can be even more severe. Smoking in pregnancy can cause a woman to miscarry or have a stillbirth. Mothers who smoke in pregnancy often have babies who are born too early or too small. These babies' lungs may be damaged or immature.

Using tobacco can rob your baby of the oxygen she needs. Tobacco has many chemicals. These can stick to the red blood cells. This prevents the red blood cells from carrying as much oxygen. Your baby gets all her oxygen from you. If your body carries less oxygen, she gets less, too. A lack of oxygen will harm her developing body and brain.

Cigarette smoke is still a danger after birth. Inhaling someone's cigarette smoke is called passive smoking. This smoke is called secondhand smoke. It can harm the lungs of anyone who breathes it. If people smoke around your baby, she will be more likely to have ear infections, asthma, bronchitis, or other breathing and lung problems. Exposing your baby to cigarette smoke may also greatly increase her risk of developing sudden infant death syndrome (SIDS). This is a condition in which a seemingly healthy infant dies while sleeping with no apparent cause.

Illegal Drugs

Illegal drugs, also called street drugs, are dangerous for anyone who takes them. They are the most deadly for an unborn baby whose mother uses them. Cocaine, heroin, and marijuana are illegal. So are amphetamines (speed, meth) and barbiturates.

Each time a pregnant woman takes these drugs, she risks her baby's life. She is likely to miscarry or have a stillbirth. Her baby is more likely to be born too early or too small. Illegal drugs can interfere with the baby's growth. Physical and mental disabilities can occur.

If you use drugs when you're pregnant, your baby may be born addicted. He may go through withdrawal after birth. This can be painful and traumatic for him. It is also dangerous. Your baby may have seizures or feeding difficulties. His nervous system may be affected. He may cry more and be more difficult to comfort than other babies. Still other effects of drug use during pregnancy are not seen until years later. Your child may have development and behavior problems. He may also be more likely to use drugs himself.

Medications

In pregnancy, over-the-counter (OTC) drugs can cause problems, too. These are medicines you can buy without a prescription. Only a few OTC medications can safely be used. See Figure 4-10. Acetaminophen (Tylenol) is one of these. Most have not been proven safe to use in pregnancy. Some are known to harm unborn babies. Don't use any OTC drug without your health care provider's okay. This even includes cold medicines, laxatives, and antacids.

If you take prescription medicines, check with your health care provider. Some of these drugs can also harm your baby. Your provider can help you weigh the benefits and risks. He or she can tell you whether to keep using your prescription or stop taking it until the baby is born.

X Rays

X rays are most dangerous in the first three months of pregnancy. This is when your baby's body is forming. X rays emit radiation that can cause physical disabilities in your baby. If any health care provider suggests an X ray, remind him or her of your pregnancy. Ask if the X ray must be taken right away. If not, postpone it until after your baby is born. If you do have an X ray, ask about safety. Be sure your provider shields your abdomen with a lead apron before the X ray. This will protect your baby.

Caffeine

Some studies show that caffeine raises the risk of miscarriage. Because of this, most health care providers advise pregnant women to limit caffeine

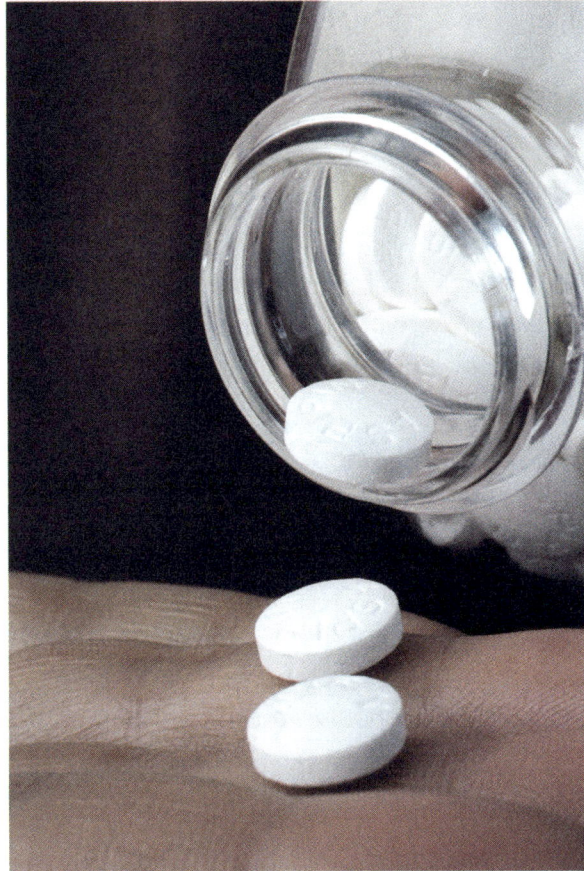

4-10 Aspirin can cause an unborn baby to bleed inside. Ask your health care provider before taking any OTC medications.

use. Many soft drinks and "energy drinks" contain high amounts of caffeine. Always check the caffeine content of the beverages. Just to be safe, you might think about cutting out caffeine. The March of Dimes suggests women have no more than one soda or one cup of coffee per day.

Exposure to Chemicals

Some chemicals can be harmful during pregnancy. A good rule is to avoid using any chemical unless it is necessary. This includes hair chemicals, such as dyes and curling or straightening agents. Paint or cleaners can create fumes. Pesticides can also be dangerous. If you're exposed to any chemical at school or work, find out the name of the substance. Your health care provider can tell you if it will harm your baby. You can protect her by avoiding exposure to chemicals.

All these guidelines can greatly reduce the risks to you and your baby during pregnancy. It will take effort, though. You may feel like there are too many rules and too much to remember. Pregnancy will only last a few months. In this time, you can do much to give your baby a healthy start. Your reward will be a healthier pregnancy and a healthier baby.

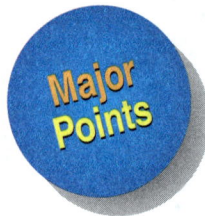

Major Points

☛ Pregnant teens and their babies are at a high risk for pregnancy complications. Teens who are younger than 15 have the greatest number of these complications.

☛ Early and regular prenatal care gives you the best chance of having a healthy pregnancy and a healthy baby. If you haven't already started prenatal care, you should do so right away.

☛ Many prenatal tests can detect possible problems with your pregnancy. You and your health care provider can decide which prenatal tests you need.

☛ The most common complications for pregnant teens are premature labor, low birthweight, anemia, preeclampsia, infections, and STIs.

☛ During pregnancy, reduce as many risks as possible to keep yourself and your baby healthy. Avoid alcohol, tobacco, and illegal drugs. Ask your health care provider about taking any medications or drinking caffeine. Stay away from radiation and chemicals.

Chapter 5
Exercising and
Eating Right

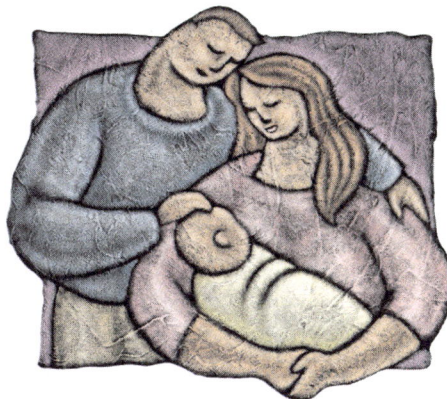

In pregnancy, you need to take care of yourself and your unborn child. Prenatal care is one way to do this. A second way is with exercise. In this chapter, you will learn how to stay fit during pregnancy. Regular exercise will keep you healthy. You will learn conditioning exercises that can help you prepare to deliver your baby.

Healthful eating is just as vital. Your body is growing, and so is your baby's. In pregnancy, you are eating to meet the nutrient needs of you and your baby. This chapter will help you choose the right kinds and amounts of nutrients. It will help you make healthful food choices.

Pregnancy and Exercise

Exercise is good for your body and emotional well-being. It is part of a healthy lifestyle. You may wonder how pregnancy affects your ability to exercise. One of your main concerns may be safety. You won't want to do anything to harm yourself or your baby. The good news is most healthy women can exercise safely in pregnancy.

Talk to your health care provider about your exercise plans. Make sure it's okay for you to do the type of exercise you had planned. (In a few cases, exercise may not be advised.) If your provider approves, try to exercise at least three times a week. Try to work out for 20 minutes or more. Ask your provider how far into the pregnancy you can exercise. Most women can exercise until close to the end of pregnancy if they feel like it.

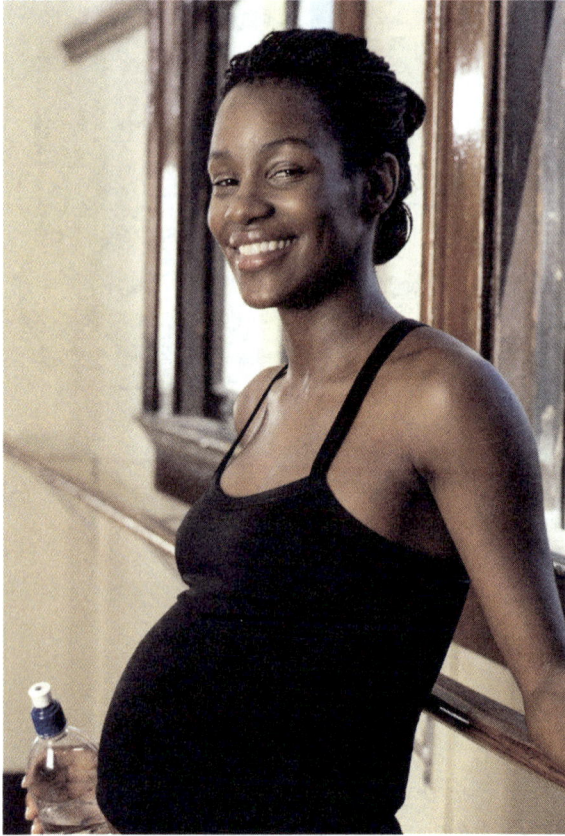

5-1 Regular exercise will help you keep your weight gain within the desired limits, which will promote a healthy pregnancy and delivery.

Regular exercise has many benefits. With regular exercise, you can do the following:

- Maintain a slow, steady weight gain. This will help you avoid gaining weight more quickly than recommended. See Figure 5-1.
- Keep your muscles toned and strong. This will help you avoid muscle and backaches.
- Feel better. Through exercise, you can relieve stress and sleep better. You'll feel more energized. You can also avoid constipation.
- Prepare for labor and delivery. If you stay active during pregnancy, your labor and delivery will be easier.
- Regain your prepregnancy shape. If you aren't active during pregnancy, you'll have more work to do after the baby is born. You'll find it harder to lose weight and rebuild your muscle tone. It will take longer to get your figure back.

Guidelines for Exercise

Exercise is good for most pregnant women. All types of exercise are not equal, though. Some are okay in pregnancy, while others are not. See Figure 5-2, which lists activities you can do and those you should avoid.

It is a good rule not to exercise much more now than before you were pregnant. Most likely, you can keep doing activities you did before your pregnancy. Don't start a new sport without asking your

Pregnancy and Exercise

Activities You Can Do	Activities to Avoid
Walking	Volleyball
Swimming/water aerobics	Basketball
Bicycling	Football
Jogging/running	Boxing/wrestling
Dancing	High intensity, high impact aerobics
Low impact, low intensity aerobics	Heavy weight lifting
Rowing	Racquetball
Tennis	Surfing/water skiing
Softball	Diving/scuba diving
Bowling	Downhill skiing
Light weight lifting	Horseback riding
Golf	Skating: ice skating, roller skating, or inline skating
Prenatal exercise classes	Mountain climbing
Pregnancy conditioning exercises	Soccer/hockey

5-2 What exercises do you like to do? Make sure your favorite isn't one you should avoid while you're pregnant.

health care provider, though. If you didn't exercise before pregnancy, you might start by walking regularly. Almost everyone can walk for exercise. Call your provider if you have any questions.

Key points about exercise in pregnancy include the following:

- Keep your pulse rate under 140 beats per minute. This will keep your body from working too hard. If you don't know how to take your pulse, ask a nurse.

- Avoid running out of breath during exercise. This is another sign you are working too hard. You should be able to talk normally while exercising.

- Include 10- to 15-minute warm-up and cool-down periods in your workouts. This helps you avoid overexerting yourself. Stretching your muscles and walking are good warm-up activities. They can also be used to cool down. As you cool down, keep moving until your heart rate is down close to normal.

☞ Be careful. Your body shape is changing. So is your sense of balance. It's also easier to injure your joints when you're pregnant.

☞ Avoid exercising in extreme weather conditions. Don't exercise outside in very hot, humid, or very cold weather. Work out indoors at these times.

☞ Do not use hot tubs or saunas. These can increase your body temperature too much.

☞ Drink fluids before, during, and after exercise to prevent dehydration.

☞ After 28 weeks of pregnancy, avoid lying flat on your back. Lying on your back could reduce the supply of oxygen to your baby. Change or stop any exercises that require you to lie on your back.

Most of the time it is fine to exercise in pregnancy. Certain signs can indicate a problem, though. Stop exercising if you notice any of the signs listed in Figure 5-3. If any of these signs occurs, let your health care provider know. He or she can make sure nothing is wrong. Your provider can also suggest a type or level of activity that may work better for you.

Warning Signs During Exercise

When exercising, stop immediately if you notice any of the following signs:

❖ dizziness
❖ numbness
❖ pain in your chest, back, hip, or pubic area
❖ trouble breathing
❖ contractions or cramps in your uterus
❖ bleeding or loss of fluid from your vagina

5-3 When you exercise, pay attention to the signals your body sends.

Conditioning Exercises

Labor and delivery are hard work. You'll push your muscles to the limit when you deliver your baby. You need strong muscles that can keep working for long periods at a time. If you prepare them, your muscles will be better able to do this work.

Conditioning is a type of exercise that makes muscles better able to do continued hard work. See Figure 5-4. Three basic kinds of conditioning exercises are useful in pregnancy. One type strengthens the muscles of the abdomen. A second type controls breathing. Third, some exercises can tone the muscles of the pelvic floor. The pelvic floor muscles support the bladder, uterus, and bowel. You use these muscles when you urinate or have a bowel movement. They also contract the vagina during sexual intercourse.

If you condition these muscles, you will regain your figure faster after childbirth. You can also prevent some other problems of the bladder, uterus, and vagina.

5-4 Conditioning exercises help your body prepare for labor and delivery. You can do them throughout pregnancy whether you're on the floor, in a chair, or standing.

The following sections explain these exercises. Detailed steps are given for each one. Do these exercises three times a week. Start with a small number of each exercise and increase gradually.

Kegel Exercise

Kegel (KEE guhl) exercise describes an exercise done by contracting and relaxing the pelvic floor muscles. This exercise is done to strengthen the muscles you will use in delivery. When you

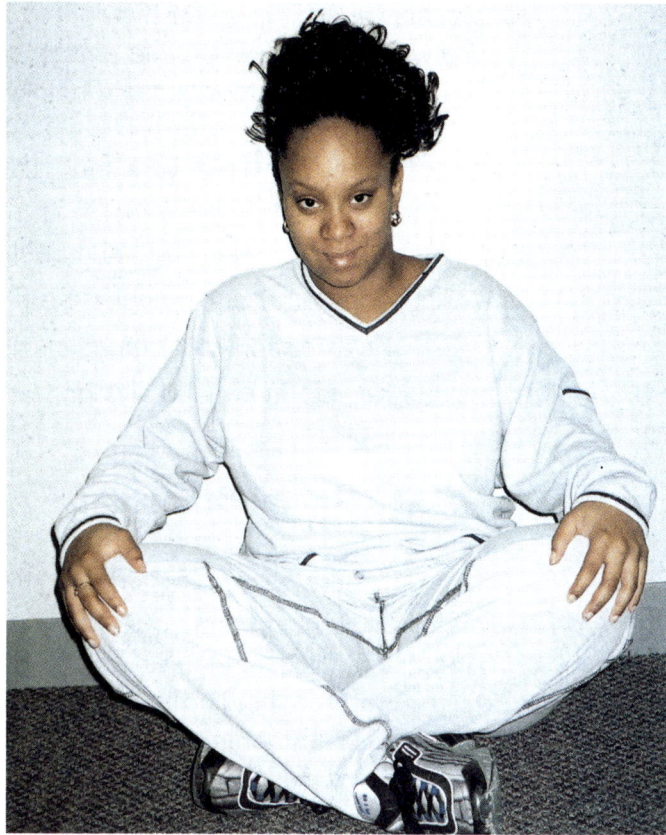

are first learning, you may wish to lie on the floor. With practice, you will find the exercise is simple to do. You can do it anywhere. To do Kegel exercises, do the following:

1. First, contract your muscles like you are holding back a bowel movement.
2. Contract your vaginal muscles.
3. Contract your muscles as if you were holding back urine.
4. Relax each set of muscles one at a time.
5. Repeat in sets of five or ten more than once a day.

Abdominal Breathing

You can work to strengthen the muscles that hold in the abdomen. Toning these muscles makes it easier to carry your baby. Abdominal breathing is an exercise that combines abdominal work with deep breathing. This deep breathing will also be helpful during labor. Good breathing techniques can help relax a woman in labor and delivery. For abdominal breathing exercises, do the following:

1. Lie on your back with your knees bent. Use this position during your first 28 weeks. After 28 weeks, lie on your side or sit in a chair or on the floor against the wall.
2. Breathe in deeply through your nose. You should feel your nostrils widen slightly.
3. Keep your ribs as still as you can. Let your abdominal wall expand upward while you are taking in the breath.
4. Then, with your lips slightly open, blow the air out slowly, but forcibly. While doing this, pull in your abdominal muscles until you have emptied your lungs.

Pelvic Tilt Exercise

The pelvic tilt exercise, shown in Figure 5-5, helps relieve backache. It conditions some of the abdominal and buttock muscles. It looks a little like a belly-dancing movement. To do this exercise, do the following:

1. Lie on your back with your knees bent. Use this position during your first 28 weeks. After 28 weeks, lie on your left side, sit in a chair, stand, or kneel on all fours. Keep your body straight.
2. Roll the pelvis back by flattening your lower back against the floor, chair, or wall. Move only your abdomen and buttocks. Imagine your upper body and abdomen are connected by a well-oiled hinge.
3. Breathe out, contracting your abdominal muscles and buttocks.
4. Hold the position for about three seconds. Relax.
5. Repeat.

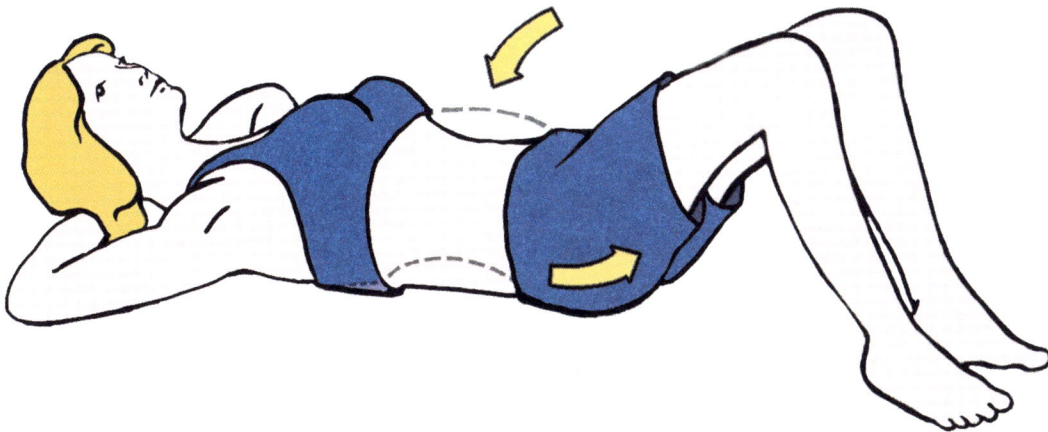

5-5 Early in pregnancy, you can do the pelvic tilt exercise lying on your back on the floor.

Leg Sliding Exercise

The leg sliding exercise also conditions some of the abdominal muscles. See Figure 5-6.

1. In your first 28 weeks, lie on your back with your knees bent. After 28 weeks, do this exercise while standing against a wall. Your pelvis should be tilted so the curve of your back is flattened against the floor or wall.
2. Hold the starting position while you slowly stretch your legs out straight. At first, you may need to do one leg at a time.
3. If your back starts to curve, slowly draw your knees up and repeat. (In time, you should be able to keep your back flat while sliding your legs out.)

Conditioning exercises like these will help prepare your body for a good childbirth experience. They will also help you feel better. Think of them as a necessary part of prenatal care. Use these exercises to take care of yourself and your baby.

Nutrition: You and Your Baby

Eating a variety of nutritious foods is vital to health. In pregnancy, you have two people to nourish—you and your baby. Getting the right amount of nutrients is important. A nutrient is a

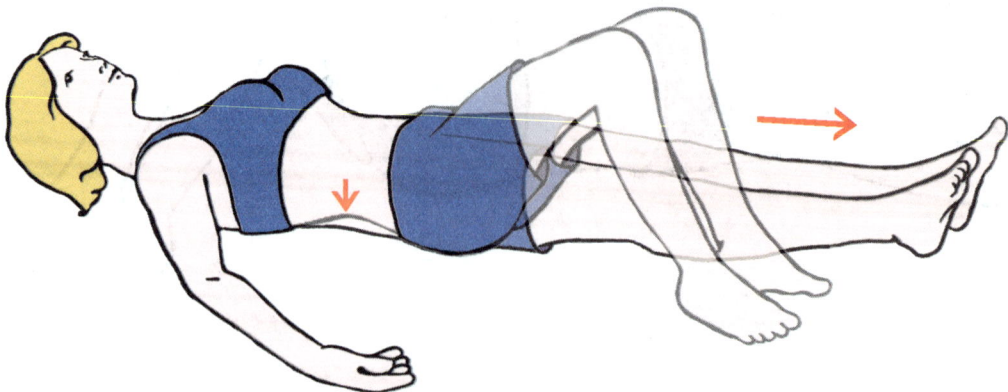

5-6 Push your lower back against the floor as you slowly straighten your legs.

chemical substance in food that helps build and maintain the body. Nutrients come from the foods you eat. They help your baby's body (and your body) grow.

Most teens don't eat all the nutrients they need. Some make very poor food choices. Their diets may not be very healthful. Was your diet healthful before you became pregnant? Now that you're pregnant, it is more important than ever that you eat right. In fact, pregnancy motivates some women to improve their eating habits. If you want to make positive changes for yourself and your baby, learning about nutrition can be a start.

Increased Nutrient Needs

Your baby takes the nutrients he needs from your body. If you ate healthful foods before pregnancy, some of these nutrients were stored in your body. Your body and your baby will use these stored nutrients to grow. Eating healthful foods helps you keep these stores full. This gives you and your baby all the nutrients you need.

In pregnancy, your need for some nutrients increases greatly. For example, you will need more energy. In your second and third trimesters, you need about 300 extra calories a day. If you're not sure how many calories this is, talk to a dietitian. Your extra calories should come from healthful foods—not junk foods. Figure 5-7 lists major nutrients that are needed in increased amounts during pregnancy. Talk to a dietitian to learn more about meeting your nutrient needs during pregnancy.

Your provider may ask you to take prenatal vitamins. These vitamins are specially designed to help women meet the increased needs of pregnancy. Taking these vitamins can make a big difference to your baby's health. Prenatal vitamins do not replace healthful foods. Instead, they work with healthful foods to fill all your nutrient needs. If your provider suggests these vitamins, take them every day.

Liquids are also important during pregnancy. Drinking enough liquids helps you avoid dehydration and constipation. Dehydration may lead to premature contractions of the uterus. Drink at least

Key Nutrients in Pregnancy

Nutrient	Functions	Sources
Iron (Mineral)	Helps red blood cells carry oxygen. Prevents anemia.	Red meats, beans, iron-fortified breakfast cereals, prunes, raisins, spinach, and peas. Also in supplements and prenatal vitamins.
Calcium (Mineral)	Builds baby's bones and teeth. Keeps mother's bones and teeth strong.	Milk, cheese, yogurt, pudding, calcium-fortified orange juice, and some vegetables. Also in supplements and prenatal vitamins.
Folic Acid (Vitamin)	Helps prevent severe disabilities of the brain and spinal cord. Builds red blood cells.	Whole-grain products, leafy green vegetables, and beans. All women of childbearing age should take a supplement containing folic acid.

5-7 The demand for these nutrients increases dramatically in pregnancy. Make sure you are getting enough of these important vitamins and minerals.

eight 8-ounce glasses of liquids a day. If you have constipation, increase your fluid intake to 10 glasses daily. During warm or hot weather, you may need even more liquid. To meet these needs, you can carry water with you when you are away from home.

Water, milk, and fruit or vegetable juices are the best liquids. Avoid fluids that contain caffeine. These include coffee, tea, and most soft drinks. Many carbonated and sweetened drinks are high in sugar but provide very few nutrients. Limit these—they don't offer anything good for you or your baby.

MyPyramid

MyPyramid is a personalized system that helps you plan a nutritious diet. MyPyramid has six triangles that stand for the five major food groups plus oils. See Figure 5-8. It encourages healthier food choices and daily physical activity. Access it at www.MyPyramid.gov. To the left of the Web page, click on Pregnancy & Breast-feeding. There you will find the section of MyPyramid designed just for you. First, it advises you to contact your health care provider to make sure both you and your baby are healthy.

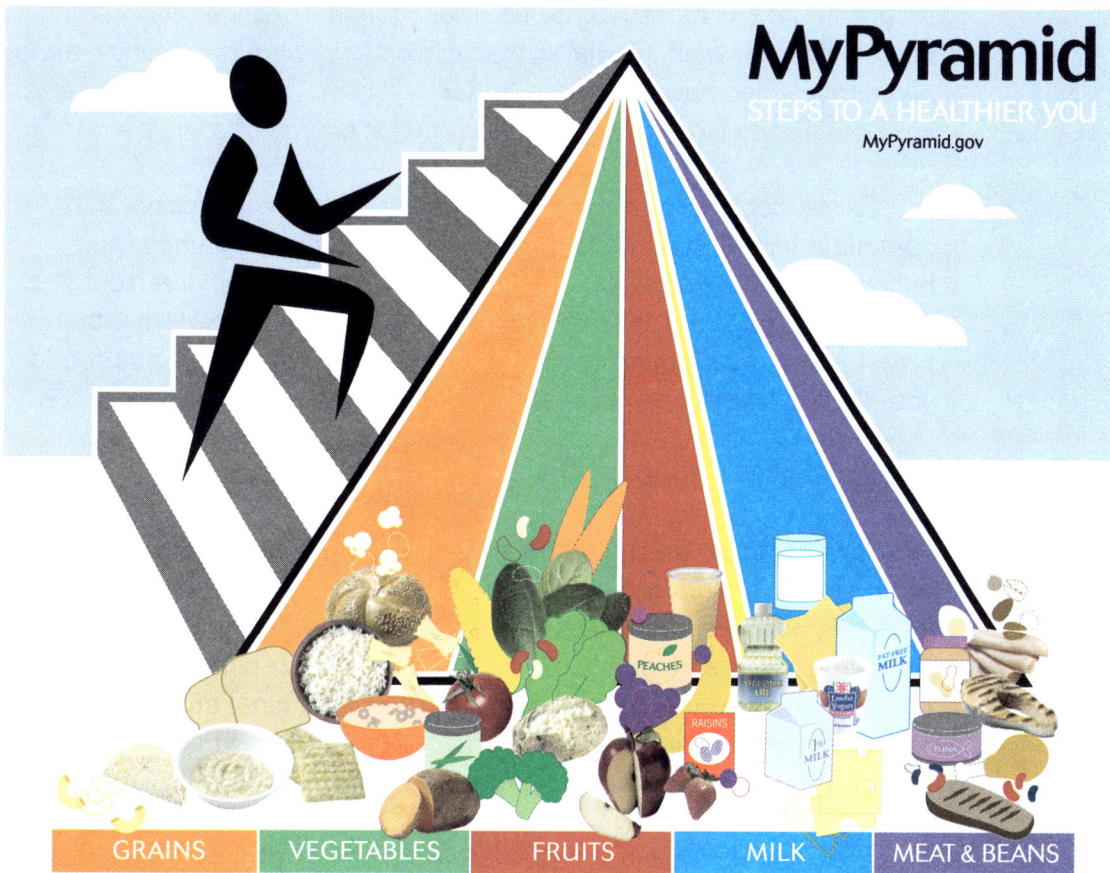

5-8 Examine this MyPyramid illustration and visit *MyPyramid.gov.* Are you eating the right types and amounts of food for you and your baby?

To get your own <u>MyPyramid Plan for Moms</u>, click on the link provided. It will ask you for information such as whether you are pregnant or breast-feeding, your age, your due date, your height, your prepregnancy weight and the amount of time you are physically active per day. Once you have entered your information, you will get an estimate of what and how much you need to eat. This will show you the foods and amounts that are right for you based on the information you provided.

Grains Group

The orange triangle of MyPyramid includes foods made from grains. Some examples of foods in this group are breads, cereals, rice, pasta, crackers, tortillas, grits, and couscous. Whole-grain products are the most nutritious. These foods are good sources of starch, fiber, thiamin, riboflavin, niacin, folic acid, and iron. Many breads and cereals also have nutrients added to them. These foods are called enriched. Foods from this group are a major source of energy.

Cakes, cookies, and pastries are also made from grains, but contain added fat and sugar. They have less fiber, vitamins and minerals than other foods in this group. The best choices from the grains group are made from whole grains, such as whole wheat bread and pasta, popcorn, and oatmeal. At least half of the foods you choose from this group should come from whole-grain sources.

Vegetable Group

The vegetable group is the green triangle in MyPyramid. Some of the foods in this group include tomatoes, broccoli, carrots, corn, cabbage, peppers, potatoes, bok choy, onions, and green beans. Others are beets, cucumbers, mushrooms, okra, spinach, and pea pods. Vegetables are a rich source of fiber, vitamins, and minerals. They differ in the kinds and amount of vitamins and minerals they provide. This is why you should eat a variety of vegetables.

The best choices of vegetables are fresh or plain frozen vegetables. Canned vegetables are often high in sodium. Also, vegetables that are fried or have a sauce are high in sodium and fat.

Fruit Group

The red triangle in MyPyramid is the fruit group. Examples of fruits are apples, bananas, blueberries, kiwifruit, oranges, pears, and papayas. Fruits are an excellent source of fiber, vitamins, and minerals. Different types of fruits contain different nutrients. For this reason, it is wise to eat a wide variety.

Fresh fruits are the best choices. They provide the most fiber, vitamins, and minerals. Cooked or canned fruits are also good, but try to avoid those cooked or packed in heavy syrup. Dried fruits are also a good choice. For the most nutrients, choose 100 percent fruit juice instead of punches, ades, and most fruit drinks. Keep the amount of fruit juice to less than half of your total fruit intake.

Milk Group

The blue triangle in MyPyramid is the milk group. Foods in this group include milk, yogurt, cheese, ice cream, and pudding. This group supplies the mineral calcium, as well as other vitamins and minerals. The milk group also offers protein, a nutrient involved in building and repairing cells. What if you can't tolerate dairy products or simply don't like them? Ask your health care provider or a dietitian what to do. You may be advised to take calcium supplements or antacid tablets that contain calcium. There are other products to use if dairy products upset you.

Whole milk and milk products contain a lot of fat. Reduced fat, low-fat, and fat-free milk and milk products are better choices. It's also a good idea to go easy on milk desserts and chocolate milk because of the added sugar.

Meat and Beans Group

The purple triangle in MyPyramid is the meat and beans group. Examples of foods in this group are beef, pork, chicken, turkey, fish, beans, eggs, nuts, and peanut butter. If you are a vegetarian (person who does not eat meat), you can still get protein from lentils, refried beans, black-eyed peas, soybeans, and tofu. This group supplies protein vitamins, and minerals.

Some meats and meat alternates are very high in fat. Try to limit these high-fat choices. Instead, choose leaner cuts of meat as well as more poultry (without the skin), and beans. Try to choose more fish, nuts, and seeds because of healthy fats they contain.

Oils

The thin yellow triangle in MyPyramid is the oils group. Oils are liquid at room temperature. They come from plants and fish. Canola, corn, olive, soybean, and sunflower oils come from plants. Oils are used in cooking and to make foods such as margarine, salad dressings, and mayonnaise. Foods that belong to other groups also add oil to your diet. These foods include nuts, olives, some fish, and avocados.

Because oils are rich in calories, go easy on oils or foods containing high amounts of them. Choose foods that are rich in unsaturated fats. One type, Omega-3 fat, is important to your health.

Making MyPyramid Work for You

Understanding MyPyramid is a good first step. Learning serving sizes can help you make sure you're eating the right amount of each kind of food. Being informed is important. It can only help if you put the information to use, though. The following tips may help.

Make snacks a part of your day. Many pregnant teens are hungry all the time, but soon feel full after eating only a small amount. Eating healthful snacks between meals will help. Many foods are easy to carry with you, such as peanuts, cheese, fruit, or crackers. These foods can keep you from getting hungry when you're away from home. Fresh fruits and vegetables will help with constipation. Limit pastries, doughnuts, cookies, and other high-fat foods.

Even with snacks, you will still need at least three meals a day. When you don't eat for a few hours, the level of sugar in your blood gets low. This can make you feel nauseated, tired, and lightheaded. You might get a headache three to four hours after the last time you ate. The baby also needs nutrients that come from the foods you eat. If you get full faster, you may want to eat several smaller meals.

Breakfast is an important meal. It starts your digestive system working. Many teens find it difficult to eat breakfast. Some just don't take the time. Don't skip breakfast. You and your baby need it. See Figure 5-9. If you are affected by nausea early in the day, try eating small amounts of dry foods, such as toast or crackers, before getting out of bed. Sometimes this helps.

When you eat in restaurants, try to make healthful food choices. Many fast foods are high in salt and fat, but low in other nutrients. You can order some healthful foods in restaurants—even fast food places. Broiled or baked meats, milk, fruit juice, salads with a little oil, baked potatoes, bagels, and lowfat muffins are some of the more nutritious items to look for in fast food restaurants. Try eating at home more often while you're pregnant. This gives you more control over what you eat.

Healthful eating is one of the best things you can do for your baby during pregnancy. You don't have to give up all your favorite foods. You just have to plan how to get the nutrients you and your baby need.

Where You Can Find Help

For many pregnant teens, money is an issue. A pregnant teen may not have enough money to buy the healthful foods she needs. In this case, she might be able to qualify for food stamps through her local public aid office. In some states, food stamps come in the form of booklets. Each food stamp is printed with a set dollar amount. This booklet can be taken to the store and used just like money to buy groceries. (Nonfood items cannot be bought with food stamps.) Many states now use an electronic card for food stamp purchases. This card looks like a debit or credit card. Each month, the card is credited with the dollar amount of food the person can buy.

The federal government also funds a program called the Special Supplemental Nutrition Program for Women, Infants, and Children (WIC). The WIC program helps pregnant or breast-feeding women and their children get the nutritious food they need.

5-9 Breakfast is the most important meal of the day because it gets your body going.

At some WIC offices, dietitians provide health screening and nutrition counseling. Breast-feeding or nutrition classes may also be offered. One of WIC's main services is to provide food.

Many WIC programs use food vouchers that are like coupons. With these vouchers, a woman can go to a local store and pick up certain food items free of charge. The items listed on the voucher may include eggs, milk, cereal, beans, peanut butter, juice, and cheese. This help allows her to spend her money on other needed items.

Some WIC programs are now starting to use an electronic card in place of food vouchers. This card looks much like a debit card or credit card. It has a PIN number for security purposes and can be used at the grocery store. The card electronically stores data on which foods a person is allowed to get with the card.

A woman can qualify for WIC while she is pregnant or breast-feeding. After the baby is born, she can receive WIC benefits for her child. As a pregnant teen, you may be eligible for WIC even if you don't have a low income. Ask your health care provider or dietitian how to contact WIC. You can also look for the WIC number in the phone book.

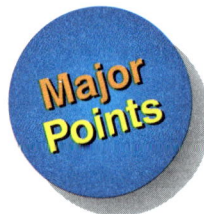

Major Points

☞ Regular exercise during pregnancy can help you to feel better both physically and emotionally. Be sure to clear your exercise plans with your health care provider. Take care to follow important guidelines and heed warnings regarding exercise.

☞ Conditioning exercises can prepare you to deliver your baby. These exercises tone and strengthen the muscles you will use in childbirth. Do these exercises three times a week or more.

☞ Eating right is one of the greatest contributions you can make to your baby's health. While you're pregnant, you will need increased amounts of certain nutrients. More of these nutrients are needed because your baby is growing and developing.

☞ If buying enough healthful food is a problem, contact your local WIC office. WIC can give pregnant women help in the form of food vouchers, nutrition counseling, and nutrition classes.

Chapter 6
Preparing for
the New Arrival

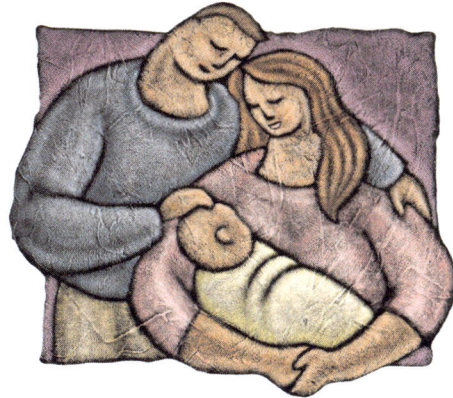

Pregnancy is a time to start making plans for the future. You and your baby's father will be parents. This is true whether you are together or not. In the months ahead, the two of you have a lot to figure out. Some of the decisions concern how you will prepare for the birth of your baby. Others involve how you will care for your baby once she is born. Both you and the baby's father must decide how you will handle school, work, parenting, and child care.

Make as many of these decisions as you can before the baby is born. You will have enough to adjust to once your baby comes. Having some choices already made will make your transition to life as a young parent easier. This chapter describes some of these issues. It will help you explore these issues and reach the decisions that are best for all of you.

Making Plans

At first, you may feel overwhelmed by your pregnancy. It will take time for you and your family to adjust to the idea. Before long, though, you may feel ready to start planning for the future. Your biggest question may be how the pregnancy will change your life. Decisions about the pregnancy take a lot of time and thought. The following sections describe four questions you might ask yourself as you start making plans.

Will I Parent or Plan an Adoption?

If you've decided to continue your pregnancy, you face another decision. This decision is whether to parent your child or make an adoption plan. For some, this is the hardest choice to make. Others know right away which option they will choose. No one answer is right for everyone. Only you can decide what's best for you and your child.

Talk to your family about your options. Your parents can help you think through this tough decision. Most likely, their reaction matters to you and you want their support. Many parents offer their love and support no matter what their pregnant teen decides. Others do not respond as well. What's important is that you try to include your family. The final decision is yours, however.

Your health care provider or a social service agency can help you choose an adoption agency. Look for an agency that will provide support and counseling for you. The agency should help you during your pregnancy and after the adoption.

If you plan an adoption, you will face different decisions from those who parent. For instance, you will need to decide the following:

- Will you choose the adoptive parents for your child?
- Do you want to see and hold your baby after she is born?
- Do you want the adoptive parents to visit at the hospital? Would you prefer the agency take the baby to the adoptive parents after you leave the hospital?
- Do you want to keep in touch with the adoptive family? (In an open adoption you would, but in a closed adoption you wouldn't.)

Two other books in this series contain information about adoption. To learn more about planning an adoption, see Understanding Your Changing Life. To learn more about the legal aspects of adoption, see Building Your Future.

What Do I Need to Do to Stay in School?

No matter which path you choose, staying in school is crucial. See Figure 6-1. Your education is valuable. It will help you turn your future plans into reality. Without a high school education, it will be hard to find a job that pays enough to support you (and your baby, if you parent).

Being pregnant makes going to school harder. At times, you may not feel well enough to concentrate on your studies. Your mind may be full of concerns about the pregnancy. Nausea and vomiting may keep you at home some days. At night, you may feel too tired to study. You may struggle to keep up with your work. There is no doubt school will be a bigger challenge than before you were pregnant.

You can succeed, but it will take effort. You will need a plan. If your pregnancy goes smoothly, it will be much easier to stay in school. It will be harder if complications occur. For instance, suppose your health care provider advises bed rest. This means you will spend a few weeks or months in bed. You would need to work with your school to arrange some way to complete your work.

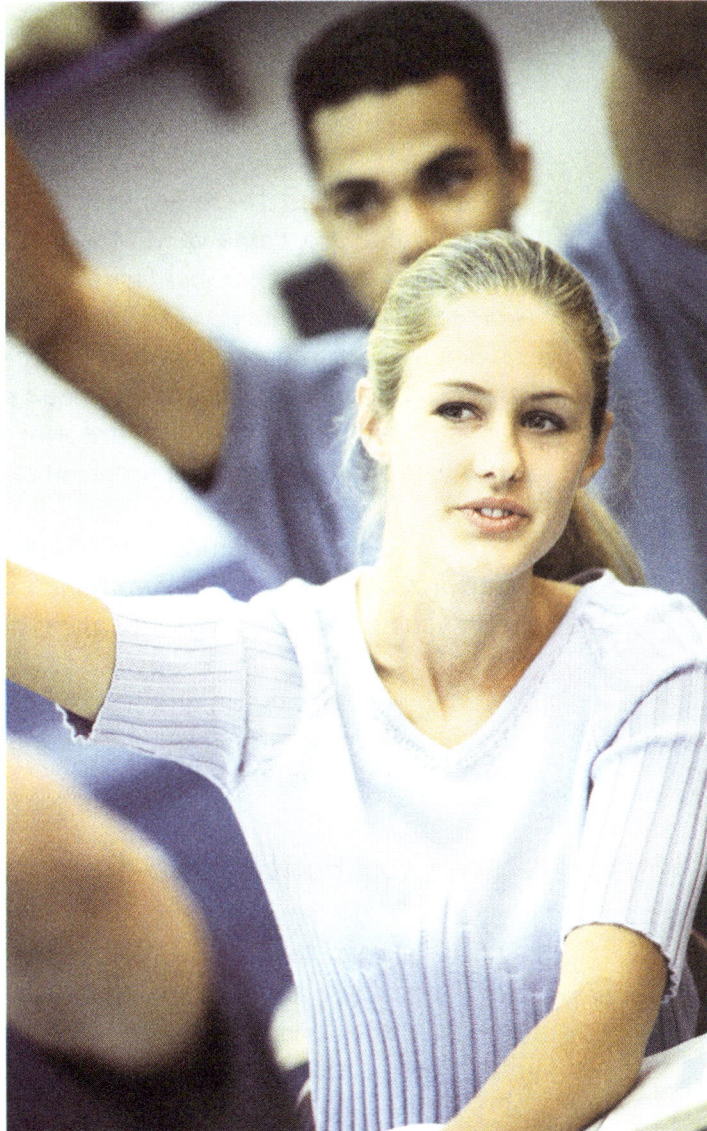

6-1 Doing whatever it takes to stay in school is a wise choice for you and your baby.

Keeping your school informed is very important. Talk to your teachers, school nurse, and guidance counselor about your situation. The school cannot work with you if they don't know what your needs are. If your school isn't cooperating with you, talk to your parents. They may be able to help you talk to the administrators.

Your teachers and guidance counselor can help you set up a plan to keep up with your studies. The options depend upon what resources your school district has. In some schools, you might be eligible for a tutor who could visit you at home. Other schools might arrange to have someone drop off and pick up your work.

In some cities, there are special school programs for pregnant teens. These programs vary. Most operate within high schools, but some are held in other locations. Some programs serve young women only while they are pregnant. After delivery, these teens return to their regular schools. Other programs serve both pregnant and parenting teens. These programs may offer child care, too. Find out what programs are available. Then you can decide whether to enter a special program or stay at your regular school.

Talk to your health care provider about your school activities. Your provider can tell you if you should avoid any of these activities while you're pregnant. For instance, he or she may write a note excusing you from unsafe gym activities. Working with chemicals in a chemistry class might also be risky. If you played any contact sports before your pregnancy, you should avoid them until after the baby comes.

What About a Part-Time Job?

The answer to this question will vary from one person to another. Some teens are already working when they find out they're pregnant. Others start working part-time while they're pregnant. These teens may want to save money for the expenses the baby will bring.

If you work during pregnancy, be sure your job doesn't harm your baby. For example, do not work with any chemicals or lift heavy objects. If your job is safe, ask yourself the questions in Figure 6-2.

Considering Work During Pregnancy

Use the following questions to help you decide whether working while you're pregnant is right for you:

❖ **How will this job affect my pregnancy?** Just as pregnancy makes school harder, it can make working harder. If you work too many hours and go to school, you may exhaust yourself. Standing for several hours can be tiresome during pregnancy. Make any needed changes in your work to protect yourself and your baby.

❖ **How will my employer and I deal with pregnancy-related absences?** At times, you may need to miss work for pregnancy-related reasons. On some days, nausea and vomiting may prevent you from working. You may have doctor's appointments. Complications may keep you from work for several weeks.

❖ **Can I work after the baby is born?** On one hand, working will bring in money you need. On the other hand, someone must care for your baby while you work. If you pay for this care, it might cost more than you make. Another concern is whether you can juggle parenting, school, and working. That's a lot to handle. With enough support from family and friends, you may be able to do it, though. Look at your situation and make the best decision for both you and your baby.

❖ **What leave will I take when the baby is born?** When the baby is born, plan to take some time off work to rest and recover. If all goes well, you might be able to return to work within a couple of weeks if you want to. If you can, you might want to take longer. You may need to spend this extra time getting to know your new baby. Talk to your employer about your company's maternity leave policy. Then you can make your decision.

6-2 Think carefully about whether working during pregnancy is right for you.

What Will I Do About Child Care?

Your baby is very precious to you. You will want to be sure he is in good hands when you return to school or work. This area is one in which parents struggle quite a bit. You won't want to leave your baby with just anyone. It takes a special person to provide daily care for a baby.

You may feel you trust people you know more than a private child care provider or a center. When you're pregnant, many relatives may offer to watch your baby for you sometime. They may be willing to provide care every now and then. This kind of care is babysitting, or care that lasts a few hours on a single day. It's a good way to meet occasional needs—when you have an appointment or just need a few hours to yourself.

Arranging this kind of care may not meet your everyday needs. Your relatives have good intentions, but they also have their own lives and responsibilities. Many times, when you need someone to care for your baby, no one may be available. Relying on this kind of care may cause you to miss enough school to fail or enough work to lose your job. It can also be stressful for you to match schedules with several different people.

What may work best is for you to find one person to take care of the baby regularly. This person might be a family member, such as your mother, aunt, or grandmother. It could also be a relative of your baby's father. You may have a relative or friend who runs a family child care home.

You may be able to think of other creative solutions to meet your child care needs. Perhaps you know a family who needs child care for their baby. If your schedules are different, maybe you could provide child care for each other. For instance, you might keep their baby in the evenings and weekends. The other family could keep your baby during the day while you're at school. This would be more work on your part, but you would save the money you'd otherwise spend on child care. That alone might make it a good option for you. As long as your child will be safe and receive good care, this is more important than who provides the care.

If a relative or friend cannot care for your baby, you may want to explore using a child care center. What's most important is that you find a good child care situation for your baby. Both you and your baby need to be happy with this arrangement. Choose your child care provider carefully. It may take you some time to find the best arrangement, so start early. You can look for the right person throughout your pregnancy. (See another title in this series, Helping Your Child Grow and Develop, for more information about child care options.)

The Baby's Father

Your baby's father is an important person in her life. This is true whether he's very involved with your pregnancy or wants no part at all. Your baby has only one father. His presence or absence in her life will affect her in big ways.

Each situation varies. You may be very close to your baby's father. He might be your husband or boyfriend. The two of you might be deeply in love and committed to parenting together. On the other hand, you might not be together. You may not speak to one another anymore. You might not even know where he is. He may not know about your pregnancy.

Many pregnant teens find themselves somewhere between these two extremes. No matter what your situation is, you play a big role in the father-child relationship. You may be able to do some of the following:

- Help him understand his roles and responsibilities as a father and a parent.
- Allow him to be involved with his child.
- Encourage him to be a good father and support his positive efforts.
- Work with him as a parenting partner.

What you cannot do is make decisions for him. You can't force him to be involved, nor can you force him out. He has rights as a father, but he must decide whether to exercise them. You aren't responsible for his relationship with your child. That's his responsibility. In some situations, you may worry about his involvement. If so, discuss this with your parents and perhaps with a lawyer. A lawyer can advise you whether to involve the court. Suppose the baby's father has a history of being abusive. You might want the court to offer only supervised visitation. (See another title in this series, Understanding Your Changing Life, for more information about your relationship with the baby's father.)

Young Dads: Roles and Responsibilities

Creating a child is much easier than being a father. See Figure 6-3. A good father takes responsibility and helps to raise his child. He provides emotional and financial support for him. A good father is committed to being an active parent in good and bad times. He is a consistent part of his child's life. He shows his love and guides his child. Dropping by once in a while is not the way to be a good father. Neither is dropping out of the picture totally.

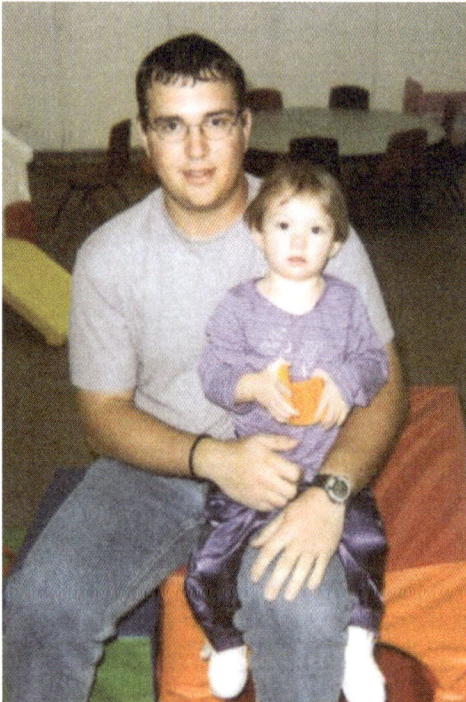

Jason Fulton, Artesia High School

6-3 Being a father is an important job. It requires commitment, effort, and dedication.

Involvement with His Child

Ideally, a father will be involved in his child's life no matter what his relationship is with the child's mother. In reality, though, things can get sticky in this area. Much depends on the relationship of the parents-to-be. If they love each other and live together, they may find it easier to agree on how they will raise their child.

More often though, the teen mother and young father have a less stable relationship. They may be certain they won't stay together. They may not live in the same house. In this case, they must discuss how the baby's father will stay involved with his child.

How does this relate to your situation? Look carefully at your relationship with your baby's father. How involved do you want him to be? How involved does he want to be? Talk to him about it if you can. Try to reach an answer to the following questions:

- ☞ How involved will he be during the pregnancy?
- ☞ Will he be present during childbirth? If so, what is his role?
- ☞ When will he see the baby? How often?
- ☞ Will he sometimes take the baby to his house?

A father-to-be can be involved right from the start. In pregnancy, he can play an important role. He can support his pregnant partner. Many pregnant teens find it hard to make lifestyle changes. In pregnancy, some of these changes are needed for the baby's health and well-being. A partner's emotional support and understanding can make these changes easier. If both partners smoke, they could quit together. (This would also make a healthier environment for the baby after birth.) He could exercise with her or cook her healthful foods. The father-to-be can attend prenatal and childbirth classes with her. He can help her during labor and participate in the delivery.

Pregnancy is the time when you and your baby's father can start to develop a relationship with your baby. Listening to the baby's heartbeat during a prenatal exam makes you feel closer to her. Parents-to-be become attached to their baby by learning the baby's activity pattern. They soon discover to which sounds or movements the baby responds. Your baby can hear some sounds, especially music, from the uterus. She might respond to music by moving. The baby becomes attached to the voices most often heard. Right after birth a baby will turn toward a familiar voice over a strange one.

After the baby is born, the father may step up and fulfill his parenting role. It is also possible he will not. If he wants to be involved, work with him for the sake of your child. Allow him to help you parent this child you created together. Think of yourselves as a team whose goal is to raise a happy, healthy child. For now, you can discuss what his role will be and whether he wants to be involved. Encourage him to establish paternity and set up visitation.

Financial Support

A father cannot deny his responsibility to support his child financially. Even if he isn't involved in any other way, he owes this to his child. Both of you created this baby, and you both have an obligation to pay your child's expenses.

You and your baby's father need to discuss money. It takes a lot of money to raise a baby. The two of you will be responsible for meeting your child's needs. You need to find out how much money you will need and where it will come from. Talk with your parents or other adults about finances.

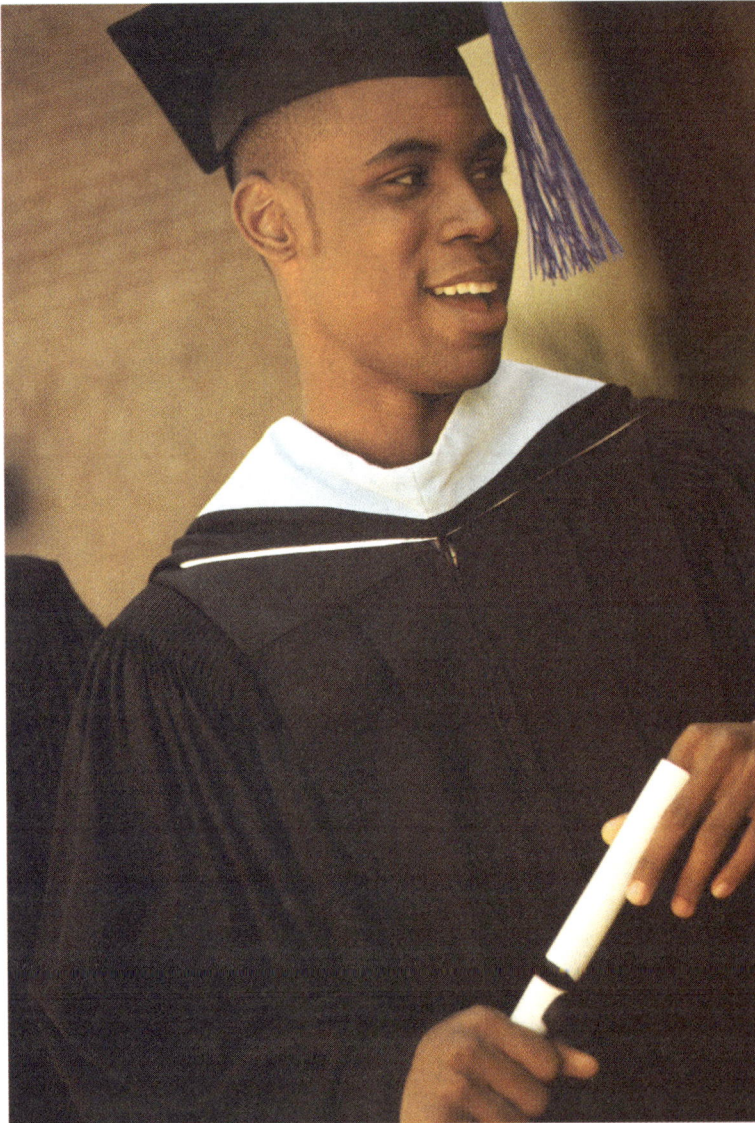

If you can live with your parents or other relatives, this will help you save money. Housing can be very costly. Your baby will also need food, clothes, and medical care. You may be eligible for some financial aid through your public aid office. Ask your health care provider, social worker, or school nurse to refer you to that office. Then you can find out if you qualify for any type of aid.

For most teens, it is not a good idea to quit school to work more hours. Your chances of getting a better-paying job improve with more education. See Figure 6-4. Most likely, you both will need to work part-time to provide some of the things the baby will need.

6-4 Graduating from high school puts teen fathers in the best position to provide financial support for their children.

What if the baby's father won't cooperate? The court can order your baby's father to pay child support for his child. If you go to court, the judge will set an amount for child support. This amount is based on your income, the father's income, and the situation. This amount must be paid each month. It may sound very simple, but often this is not the case. For instance, suppose the young man denies being the baby's father. Tests must be done to prove whether the child is his. Then the judge can rule about support. In some states, a teen father's parents can be ordered to pay support if their son has no income. To take legal action, talk to a lawyer or the legal aid society about your options. (You can read more about these legal matters in another title in this series, Building Your Future.)

Role Models for Young Dads

During pregnancy, young fathers-to-be start to wonder what kind of parents they will be. Parenting doesn't come naturally. Most people learn this role from other parents—usually their own.

Some young men have male relatives, such as grandfathers, uncles, and cousins who set an example for them. These people are called role models. A role model is a person whose actions are copied by others. Through actions, a role model sets an example that others might follow.

A young dad might admire another father for the way he relates to children. This person would be a role model for fatherhood. Many young fathers do not have adult male role models in their homes. They may not know their fathers, uncles, or grandfathers very well. Other men might serve as role models for these young fathers. Possible role models might be teachers, religious leaders, youth group leaders, or athletic coaches.

Some cities are developing programs for young fathers. These programs may be part of a teen mothers' program or they may be separate. Some are part of youth groups. The purpose of most of these groups is to provide support and parenting role models for young fathers.

Choosing Baby's Health Care Provider

During your pregnancy, take time to choose a health care provider for your baby. It's best to make this choice before the baby is born. This way, the provider can care for him just after birth. The baby will also need an appointment when he is one to two weeks old.

You might take your baby to a pediatrician. This is a doctor who specializes in caring for babies and children. A pediatrician treats only children and knows parents' concerns quite well. This kind of doctor can be a good choice.

Family practice doctors can also provide good care. They specialize in treating families. Your baby's provider might be located in a private office or in a clinic.

- Ask for recommendations. Friends or relatives may know a good provider. Your own provider may be able to suggest someone. Some cities or towns offer special medical services for the children of teen parents. Your school counselor or nurse should know if there are any of these services in your area.
- Choose a convenient location. You may need to take your baby to the doctor or clinic often. Babies need quite a few regular checkups. They also need medical care when they are sick. If you don't drive, select a place you can get to easily. You might need to walk, use public transportation, or arrange a ride.
- Ask about payment arrangements. Does the provider accept your insurance or Medicaid? What are the charges for office visits? Can these be billed?

Deciding What You Will Feed the Baby

Choosing a feeding method for your baby is a big decision. You'll want to give this decision some thought. You may not be sure until the baby comes. If you learn about both options, though, it will help. Then you'll be prepared to decide when the time comes.

Breast Milk Versus Formula

You can feed your baby breast milk, formula, or both. For some, this is a tough decision. Others seem to know right away which option they will choose. Learning about your options may help you decide. Find out about both options even if you think you know which you will use. That way you'll be informed if you should happen to change your mind.

Experts strongly support breast-feeding (also called nursing) as the best choice for most newborns. Your body was designed to make milk for your baby. Breast milk is the perfect food for your baby. It contains all the nutrients your baby needs to support her growth. Breast milk is easier for your baby to digest than formula. This means she will have less gas, diarrhea, and constipation than if you fed her formula.

Breast milk also has many other benefits for your baby. It contains antibodies, or substances that help the body fight disease. These antibodies can help your baby stay healthy. Infants who are fed breast milk have lower rates of many illnesses than formula-fed babies. See Figure 6-5. The skin-to-skin contact between you and your baby promotes her emotional growth. It makes her feel loved and secure. Studies have also shown infants who breast-feed rate higher in intellectual growth and do better in school.

Advantages of Breast Milk

	For Baby	For Mother
Breast milk reduces the chance of...	diarrhea, gas, and constipation sudden infant death syndrome (SIDS) meningitis allergies and asthma ear infections and colds pneumonia, wheezing, and bronchiolitis, diabetes other illnesses	osteoporosis breast cancer ovarian cancer
Breast milk promotes...	easier digestion better health and immunity to illness brain growth and development social and emotional development parent/child attachment less unnecessary weight gain	quicker return of body to its prepregnant state weight loss parent/child attachment financial savings over infant formula

6-5   Breast-feeding has many advantages for mothers and their babies.

In addition, breast-feeding your baby has many benefits for you. Nursing causes your body to release certain hormones. Some of these hormones help you feel relaxed and calm. Others help your uterus contract and return to its normal size. This will help you regain your figure faster. It takes many calories for your body to produce breast milk. This can promote weight loss. Breast-feeding can also lower your risk of developing bone disease and cancers of the ovaries and breasts later in life. Feeding your baby breast milk will save you a lot of money because infant formula is expensive. It can also build your confidence as a mother and increase your loving feelings toward your baby.

You can discuss nursing with your health care provider or a lactation consultant (professional who teaches women about breast-feeding). Another idea is to call a local chapter of La Leche League, an organization that supports breast-feeding. (Leche means milk in Spanish.) If you know women who have been successful with breast-feeding, you might also ask them for advice.

Some teens are concerned that breast-feeding around others will be embarrassing. They have concerns about modesty. With a little practice, you can learn to nurse without feeling exposed. You can use a blanket to cover the baby while she is eating. Choosing the right clothing can also help.

You might think you can't keep nursing your baby when you return to work or school. This is not true. Breast milk can be expressed (pumped from the breast) and fed to a baby in a bottle. This can also give others, such as the father, a chance to feed her, too. You can also nurse her in the morning, in the evening, and on weekends.

It is not recommended to start the bottle right away. For the first few weeks after your baby is born, it is best to use only breast-feeding. The baby needs to learn how to use her jaws to get milk from the ducts of the breast. Also, your body needs to build a good supply of milk. After a few weeks of nursing, it is okay to introduce a bottle. If your baby is like most babies, she will soon learn to do both.

A few women are advised not to feed their breast milk to their babies. One reason this might happen is if the mother has an illness that might enter the breast milk and harm the baby. For instance, HIV can be passed in breast milk. A woman with HIV would be advised not to breast-feed her baby. Women who take certain medications may also be advised not to feed their babies breast milk. Talk to your health care provider if you have concerns about whether your breast milk is safe for your baby.

Instead of breast milk, a woman may decide to feed her baby an infant formula. A good infant formula can supply all the nutrients your baby needs. However, it can't give her antibodies. If you will feed your baby formula, ask her health care provider which one to use. This formula will probably be iron-fortified, which means iron has been added.

Using Both Breast Milk and Formula

Many women feed their babies both breast milk and formula. This gives their babies the benefits of breast milk. It allows mothers the convenience of using formula at some times. If you want to use both breast milk and formula, talk to your health care provider or a lactation specialist. This person will advise you how to do this without limiting your breast milk supply.

What if you're not sure which method to use? Give breast-feeding a try. After trying it, you can always switch to the bottle if you choose. The opposite is not true. If you don't breast-feed right away, your milk will dry up. You will lose the chance to use this method.

It's important to choose the feeding method you find most satisfying. If you're pleased, your baby will feel good about eating. He needs nourishment, love, and attention at feeding time. You can provide these emotional benefits no matter whether you choose breast milk or formula.

Prenatal and Childbirth Classes

During pregnancy, you may want to take special classes to prepare for labor and delivery. Prenatal classes will teach you about pregnancy. You'll learn about the changes in your body. The teacher will explain how your baby changes and grows. You will also learn how to take care of yourself during pregnancy. Some prenatal classes teach infant feeding and care.

A second type of class is a childbirth class. This class will teach you about labor and delivery. You'll learn the signs of labor, when to go to the hospital, and how a baby is born. The teacher may show you special breathing and relaxation exercises. These can help you relax and cope with the pain of childbirth. You will probably want someone to be with you during labor and delivery. This person would be your labor helper. Your baby's father, your mom, or a friend might be your helper. Childbirth classes can teach this person to help you during the birth.

If you know you will be delivering without a labor helper, taking a childbirth class will help you learn to relax. The labor nurses know the techniques and will be able to help you during delivery. Share with your caseworker, health care provider, or a counselor your feelings about delivering by yourself. This will allow you to enjoy your experience rather than focusing on feeling alone.

Ask about a doula. A doula is a person trained to be a labor supporter. Doulas usually charge for their services, but many facilities have a list of doulas who are willing to be a labor support for a teen without charging a fee.

Your childbirth class may tour the birth facilities. Once you see where you will give birth, you may feel less afraid. You might even meet the nurses who will help during the birth. See Figure 6-6.

Some agencies combine their prenatal and childbirth classes. Many agencies also provide special classes for pregnant teens. If you attend these, you can talk with someone your age who is in a situation like yours. Ask your health care provider, school nurse or counselor about classes in your area. Learning what to expect is the biggest benefit of these classes. Pregnancy and childbirth are

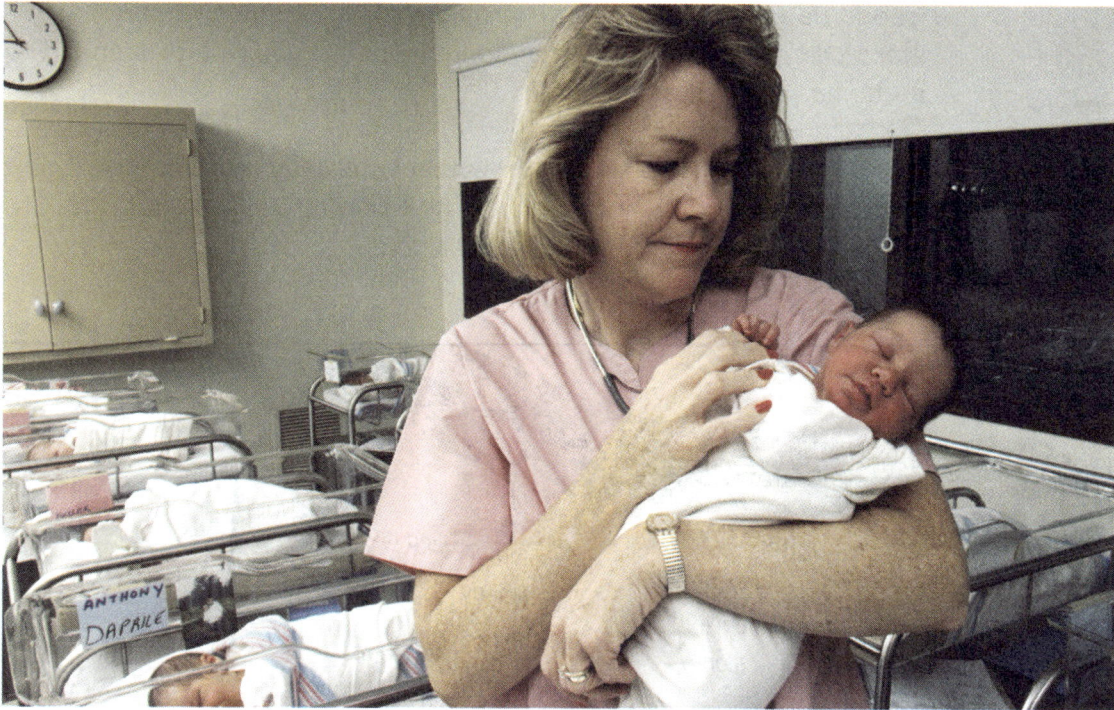

6-6 On a visit to the hospital, you might want to stop by the nursery and meet the nurses who will help you care for your newborn. This may put your mind at ease about your upcoming hospital stay.

more satisfying if you know what is happening and why. Being prepared can make it all less scary. In childbirth classes, you learn to work with your body. This may make the process go a little faster.

Planning Your Hospital Stay

As your due date draws near, you'll probably start thinking about your upcoming hospital stay. You will be at the hospital only a short time. The average stay for an uncomplicated birth is a little less than two days. Expect to stay a few days longer for a complicated delivery.

What should you pack to take with you to the hospital? You will need to have some things with you in your room. You can pack other items for when you and the baby come home. A good rule is that less is usually best. You can probably have someone bring you more things if you must stay longer or find you've left something at home. See Figure 6-7.

Plan to start packing a few weeks before the baby comes. This way you will be ready when she is! The following sections suggest what to pack for your hospital stay.

What Should You Pack?

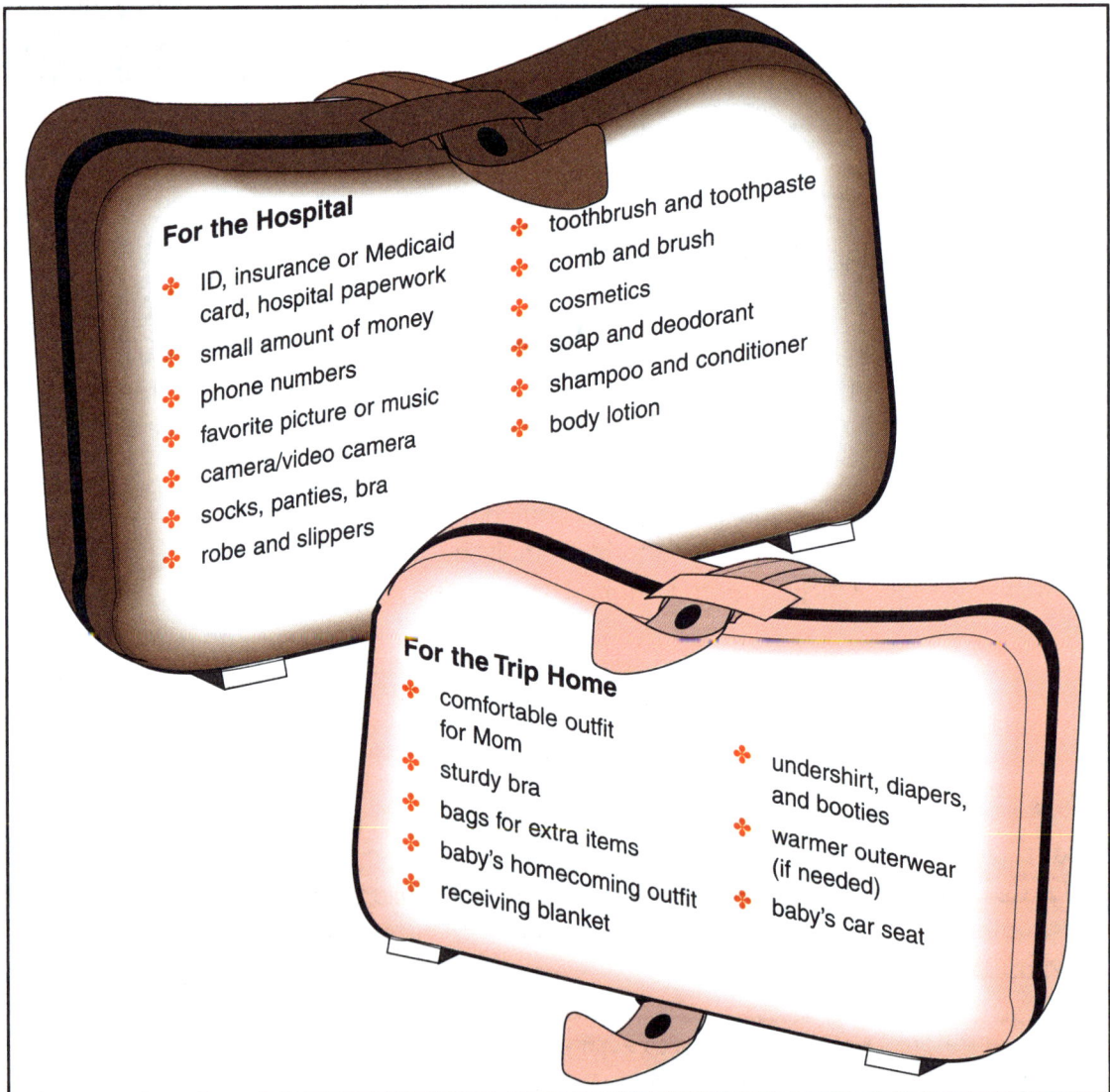

For the Hospital

- ID, insurance or Medicaid card, hospital paperwork
- small amount of money
- phone numbers
- favorite picture or music
- camera/video camera
- socks, panties, bra
- robe and slippers
- toothbrush and toothpaste
- comb and brush
- cosmetics
- soap and deodorant
- shampoo and conditioner
- body lotion

For the Trip Home

- comfortable outfit for Mom
- sturdy bra
- bags for extra items
- baby's homecoming outfit
- receiving blanket
- undershirt, diapers, and booties
- warmer outerwear (if needed)
- baby's car seat

6-7 Do you have these items "in the bag?" If not, be sure to pack them a few weeks before your due date.

What to Pack for Yourself

When you go to the hospital in labor, you will need the following items:

- ☛ ID cards, insurance or Medicaid cards, hospital paperwork.
- ☛ personal care items—toothbrush, toothpaste, comb, brush, cosmetics (if you want them), lip balm, deodorant, shampoo, conditioner, soap, and body lotion. Your hospital may provide some toiletries. If you're in doubt, ask.
- ☛ snack food—You may want to suck on hard candy while you're in labor. After the delivery, you might like to snack on dried fruit. Eating fruit can soften your bowel movements.
- ☛ a favorite picture to use as a focal point—tape this to the wall during labor. It can help you focus on breathing and relaxation techniques during contractions.
- ☛ phone numbers of people you want to call after the baby is born.
- ☛ a small amount of money and some reading material. Leave your wallet and jewelry at home. Do not bring valuables or much money.
- ☛ clothing—socks (your feet can get cold during labor), a sturdy bra, roomy panties (three or four pairs), and slippers (optional). You can take a washable robe or use a hospital gown as a robe. You may wish to wear hospital gowns instead of your own nightgowns. At night, you may sweat heavily. Plus, you won't have to worry about getting blood stains on your own clothes.
- ☛ music—If music relaxes you, ask if you can take a small battery-operated radio or personal media player with headphones.
- ☛ camera or video camera—You may want to take pictures or videotape all or parts of the birth. If so, have your labor helper take care of the camera for you. This way you will not have to worry it will be stolen or lost.

In some hospitals, a labor helper can stay overnight. If so, he or she will need to pack personal items, too. Have him or her pack pajamas, a robe, slippers, and toiletries.

In a second bag, pack the clothes you want to wear when you come home. Ask the person who will bring you home to take this bag to the hospital. Then you won't have too much to carry when you're admitted. This bag won't be in your way at the hospital. It should contain a supportive bra (nursing bra if you're breast-feeding) and comfortable clothes. Something you wore during pregnancy will be best. You probably won't fit into your regular clothes yet. Include a couple of paper or plastic bags to bring home any gifts or sample products you get while you're in the hospital.

What to Pack for the Baby

You may wonder what to pack for the baby. Basically, you just need clothes for him to wear home. This may be one of the few times he will wear newborn clothes, or those size 0-3 months. You will need the following:

- an undershirt
- diapers
- an outfit of your choice—one-piece outfits are very practical and comfortable
- booties (unless the outfit covers his feet)
- a small blanket, sometimes called a receiving blanket
- sweater and hat, heavier blankets, or a bunting, if the weather is cold

You can pack the baby's items in the same bag with your clothes to wear home. You might also want to pack a camera or video camera in this bag. Many proud parents want to take pictures of their new babies the day they come home from the hospital. You really don't need much else for the baby until after you get home. <u>Remember you must have an approved car safety seat in place for the ride home!</u>

Packing your bags for the hospital is one of the final preparations you will make. By this time, you will have spent several months getting ready for your baby's arrival. Many important decisions will already be made. This will free you to enjoy your new little one. Near the end of pregnancy, you can still make a few last-minute preparations. The wait is almost over. Soon labor will begin and your baby will be born.

☛ While you're pregnant, you have many big decisions to make. You can decide whether to parent or plan an adoption. You can make plans about school, work, and child care.

☛ A good father takes responsibility and helps to raise his child. He has important roles and responsibilities in his child's life. Young fathers can learn how to be involved with their children from other fathers, who can serve as role models.

☛ During pregnancy, you can choose your baby's health care provider. This gives you plenty of time to decide. You will not want to wait until your baby is born.

☛ Deciding how to feed your baby is an important decision. Weigh the pros and cons of each method before deciding. Choose the method that will work best for you and your baby.

☛ Prenatal and childbirth classes can help you understand pregnancy and the birth process. Knowing what to expect can prepare you for delivery. Through these classes you can also meet other pregnant teens.

☛ Pack for your hospital stay ahead of time. You will want to be prepared in case your baby comes early. Pack only what you will really need. Your stay will probably be short, so you won't need to take much with you.

Chapter 7
Experiencing
Childbirth

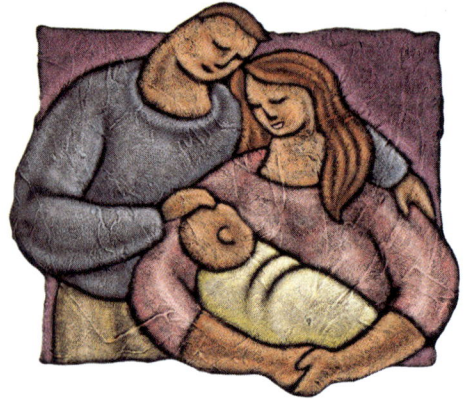

Throughout pregnancy, you've waited for the special day when your baby will be born. You've spent months preparing for this time. You have learned how to care for yourself during pregnancy. You know what exercises will condition the muscles used in childbirth. In prenatal or childbirth classes, you have studied breathing and relaxation techniques to use in labor. Your bags are packed and are ready to go. Now it's time to wait for your baby!

Mixed feelings are common at this time. Most of the time, you may feel you can't wait to see your baby. In other ways, you may not feel totally prepared for her yet. You may be excited but nervous or happy but scared. This is normal. Most parents-to-be have these feelings just before their babies are born.

Childbirth is the process through which a baby is born. Through childbirth, the baby leaves the uterus and enters the outside world. To accomplish this, a woman's body goes through labor. Labor describes the work her uterus and cervix will do to prepare to deliver the baby. Delivery describes the actual movement of the baby and the placenta from the uterus out of the body.

Childbirth can be compared to a runner preparing for a marathon. A female marathon runner eats nutritious foods to build up her body. In pregnancy, eating right helps both mother and baby become healthy and strong. A runner trains for a race with a planned program of exercise. In pregnancy, conditioning exercises will strengthen the muscles a woman will use to deliver her baby.

Running a marathon is very hard physical work. Having a baby is, too. The runner must stay focused on the goal of finishing. Marathon runners must often face pain in order to finish the race. The same is true of a woman in labor. She must keep the goal in mind—meeting a healthy baby. This will help her endure the pain.

Your childbirth experience will depend upon how well you have prepared for it. It will go best if your body is in good condition and you have a positive outlook. Labor is hard work and part of it is painful. It has a purpose, though. You are bringing your baby into the world. Staying focused on this purpose can make things easier.

This chapter describes the process of childbirth. It will explain how labor starts, and what occurs every step of the way. Knowing what to expect can calm your fears, too.

The Last Weeks of Pregnancy

Near the end of pregnancy, you will notice physical changes. These changes mean your body is getting ready for labor. For instance, you may have false labor contractions. The baby will change his position. You may notice more or different vaginal discharge, too.

False Labor

In the last few weeks of pregnancy, you may start to have some contractions. A contraction is the tightening and relaxing of the muscles of the uterus. During a contraction, you will notice your abdomen gets hard and then softens again. When you are in labor, contractions will help the uterus to open the cervix and move the baby down into the birth canal. Not all contractions are true labor contractions, however.

As your due date gets close, the uterine muscles will become very sensitive. They may contract even if labor hasn't started. These contractions are called false labor. They do not open the cervix or move the baby down the birth canal. You might also hear these contractions called Braxton-Hicks contractions.

At first, you may have a hard time telling whether a contraction is false labor or true labor. Figure 7-1 describes each type. Learning about false labor can also help you know the difference. If you're ever unsure, consult your health care provider.

Contractions: True or False Labor?

True	False
Open the cervix and move the baby down the birth canal.	Do not open the cervix or move the baby down the birth canal.
Are regular—evenly spaced and slowly growing closer together in a pattern.	Are irregular—unevenly spaced and not in a pattern of slowly growing closer together.
Build in intensity—have a pattern of getting longer and more painful as delivery nears.	Vary in intensity—do not have a pattern and may or may not be painful.
Will not stop until the baby is delivered.	May stop with fluid intake, activity, or a shower or bath. May start again a few times before labor actually begins.

7-1 Telling the difference between true labor and false labor can be tricky. When in doubt, call your health care provider.

False labor contractions vary in intensity. Some may be painful. These contractions might make your back hurt or cause pressure in your lower abdomen or vagina. At other times, contractions might feel like the cramps you may have with your periods. Still others don't hurt but cause pressure and make your abdomen feel hard. Women often describe this feeling as the baby "balling up."

If you have any contractions in the last weeks of pregnancy, don't panic. Just time them. Write down what time each contraction starts. If contractions are evenly spaced and slowly grow closer together, this may be true labor. False labor contractions are irregular—they don't have a pattern of slowly getting closer together. They often stop suddenly. True labor contractions don't stop until the baby is delivered.

You may have false contractions several times in the last few weeks of pregnancy. Some women have them on and off for the last few months. If you have these contractions, you can try several things to get them to stop. These include the following:

- ☛ drink two or three glasses of juice or water within an hour of the contractions
- ☛ take a warm shower or bath
- ☛ walk around

If any of these efforts make the contractions stop, they were false labor contractions. Call your health care provider if contractions don't stop or you're concerned. This is very important if it's earlier than week 37 of your pregnancy and you have more than four contractions in an hour. This could mean you're having premature labor. If so, you will need prompt medical attention to stop the contractions and prevent premature delivery. You may want to look back in Chapter 4 to review the warning signs of premature labor.

Baby's Position Changes

In the last few weeks of pregnancy, the baby's head will settle into the pelvic area. It will rest on top of the cervix until delivery. This is called lightening. This head-down position makes it easiest for her to enter the birth canal. After lightening happens, you will notice the following changes:

- ☛ You can breathe easier because your lungs have more room.
- ☛ The curve of your abdomen will look lower.
- ☛ The baby's head will rest on your bladder now, so you'll have to urinate more often.
- ☛ The increased pressure on your hips and pelvic bones will make it more difficult to walk.
- ☛ You will feel a lot of pressure in your birth canal.

Vaginal Discharge

As you near the end of pregnancy, you will notice more vaginal discharge. It may be clear or a little yellow in color. The discharge will be somewhat sticky. Some of it comes from the mucus plug in your cervix. In pregnancy, this mucus plug fills the cervix to keep fluids or bacteria out of the uterus. This protects your baby. When labor is near, the mucus plug is no longer needed. It starts to come out as the cervix softens and gets ready to open.

The plug may contain a little blood, so the discharge might have a light pink tint to it. This is normal. It is called the show or the bloody show. You might see this quite a few days before labor starts. It can also happen after contractions have begun. If you have any bright red discharge, call your health care provider.

Pain Relief During Childbirth

Being anxious about childbirth is normal. A little anxiety can be helpful. It keeps you alert. Fear, however, is not helpful. It can make the pain of childbirth seem much, much worse. When you're afraid, you get tense and your muscles tighten. Tense, tight muscles cause more pain during contractions. The pain can scare you, making you tense your muscles more. You can see how each step in this pattern leads to the next.

The muscles of your uterus will work better if you are not tense. The following ideas can help you prepare yourself so you won't be afraid.

- ☛ Don't let what other people say frighten you. Each birth experience is different.
- ☛ Learn about the childbirth process and what to expect. Go to classes, read books, and watch videos. See Figure 7-2. During labor, you'll be less afraid if you know what is happening and why.

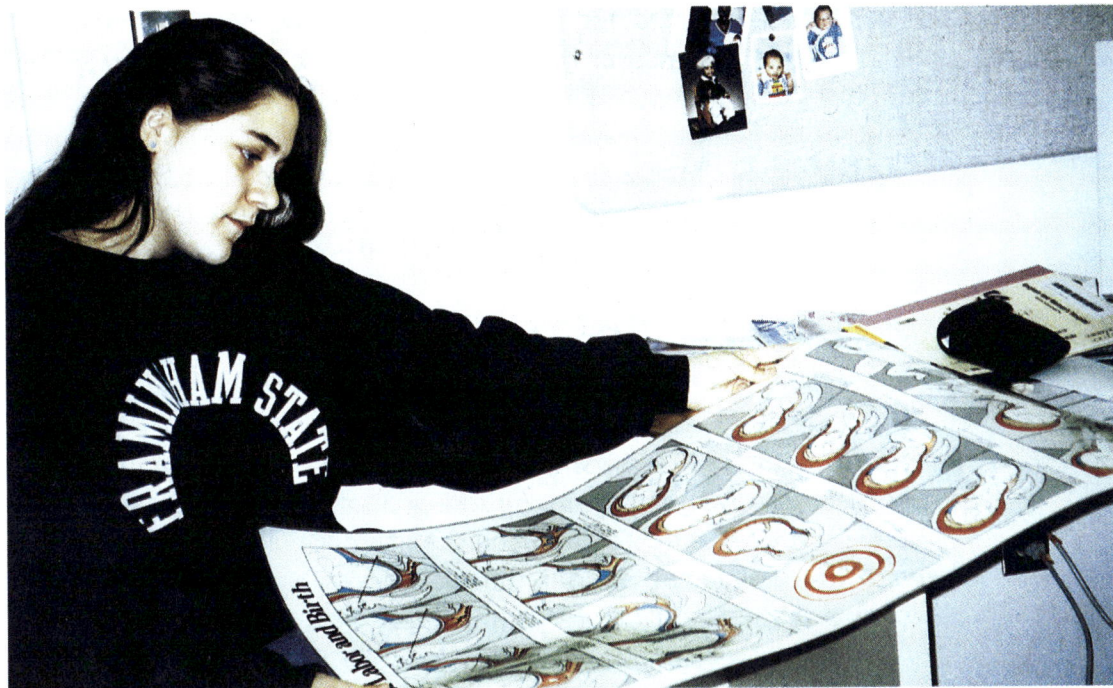

7-2 Ask your health care provider if he or she has any childbirth materials you can review. This poster shows the stages of labor.

- Learn and use breathing and relaxation exercises. These exercises will prepare you to cope with labor and delivery. Most childbirth classes include them. You can learn to work with your body so your uterine muscles will work more efficiently.
- Ask lots of questions. No question is too silly to ask!
- Keep in mind how many women have done this before! You will do fine.

In your third trimester, start thinking about what pain relief if any you will use for childbirth. Talk to your doctor or midwife about your options. Learn about all your options even if you think you know what you will do. This way you will be informed if you change your mind later.

Some women choose not to use medicine for labor. Childbirth without pain medication is called prepared childbirth. These women use breathing and relaxation exercises to cope with the pain. Their labor coaches help them focus on relaxing. If a woman doesn't use medicine, she may recover faster and be more alert. Her baby will be more alert at delivery, too.

If you'd rather not use medication, tell your health care provider. He or she can help you prepare to do this. Understanding the birth process will help you give birth without medication.

Medication for Pain Relief

Childbirth does involve some pain. Don't feel guilty if you want some medication. Many women have at least a little medication to help them deal with this pain. Anything that helps you have a safe, happy delivery is okay. You and your health care provider can talk about what medicines are safe for childbirth. Together you can choose one that best meets your needs.

Two types of medicine are used for pain relief in childbirth. Analgesia (a-nuhl-JEE-zhuh) acts on the whole body. It reduces pain and discomfort but doesn't take them away completely. An analgesic is given as a shot or intravenously (by IV). An IV is a thin tube through which liquids can travel directly into your vein. The IV would be inserted into a vein in your hand or arm. Analgesia can help you cope better with pain. During active labor, it can help you sleep between contractions.

The second type of pain relief is anesthesia (a-nuhs-THEE-zhuh), which numbs all or part of your body. There are three kinds of anesthesia. Each affects a certain area of the body. If you have anesthesia, you won't feel anything in the area where it works.

General anesthesia numbs the entire body. It is used to put you to sleep. If you don't like pain, this may sound like a great way to have a baby! Actually, this type of medicine can be dangerous for your baby. It can make him too sleepy at birth. He may not be able to breathe well. Risks exist for you, too. General anesthesia is not used often for childbirth. It is saved for emergency situations.

Regional anesthesia is the type most often used in childbirth. This medicine numbs part of the body, but doesn't make you sleep. Regional anesthesia has fewer bad effects on the baby. It may lengthen your labor, though. You won't be able to feel the contractions. This may make it harder for you to know when and how to push.

The type of regional anesthesia used most often in childbirth is an epidural (ep-ih-DUR-uhl). For an epidural, a thin tube is inserted through the covering of the spinal cord into the space around the cord. The end of this tube is taped to your back. Medicine is injected into the tube continuously. This medicine will numb you below your waist. You shouldn't feel any pain. If feeling returns, more medicine can be put through the tube. The medicine should wear off a few hours after delivery.

Local anesthesia takes away pain in a small area. It is most often injected into the area to be numbed. In childbirth, local anesthesia may be used if stitching is necessary. It is also sometimes used before a small cut is made in the birth canal to give the baby more room to be delivered.

Stages of Labor

Most births are vaginal births. In this type of birth, the baby uses the vagina (birth canal) to travel out of the mother's body. For a vaginal birth, labor includes three stages. The first stage is the opening of the cervix, which consists of three phases. The second and third stages are the delivery of the baby and the delivery of the afterbirth. At the end of labor, you will meet your baby for the first time.

With a first baby, childbirth lasts an average of 12 to 24 hours from the start of labor to the delivery of the baby and placenta. Each labor and delivery is unique. Some are very short, while others are quite long. Most are somewhere in the middle. Some women remember childbirth as a bad, painful experience. Many women say it wasn't as bad as they thought it would be. Most women remember labor as painful but satisfying. These women say the pain was worth it because it helped them have their babies.

Once labor begins, it will progress through three stages. Each stage plays a role in bringing your baby into the world.

Stage One: Opening of the Cervix

Stage one of labor lasts an average of 8 to 20 hours for a first baby. The purpose of this stage is to slowly open the cervix so your baby can come out. This is called dilatation (dihl-uh-TAY-shun). The opening of the cervix measures less than 1 centimeter (cm) before pregnancy. In labor, this opening must widen to 10 cm (about 4 inches). See Figure 7-3. The baby's head needs this much room to come out. As the cervix opens, it also gets shorter and thinner. This is called effacement (ih-FAY-smuhnt). Effacement is described as a percentage (100 percent is total effacement). In the last weeks of pregnancy, your cervix may dilate and efface a little.

Dilatation of the Cervix

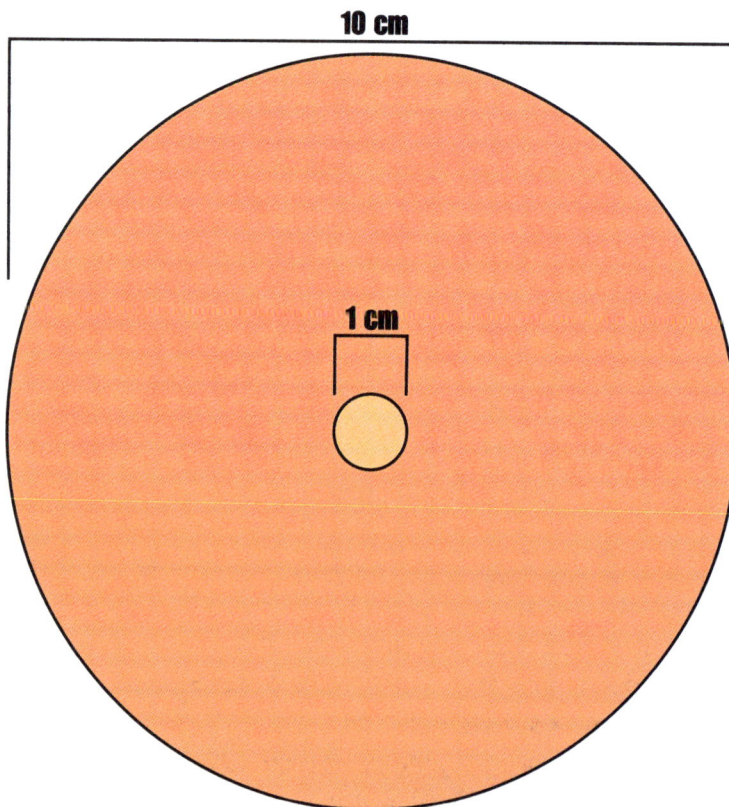

10 cm

1 cm

7-3 During labor, your cervix will dilate from less than 1 cm to 10 cm.

Early in labor, mild contractions may occur 20 to 30 minutes apart. These early contractions last only about 30 seconds. They are not painful. As your labor progresses, the tightening of your uterine muscles will gradually cause you more discomfort. Your contractions will slowly get stronger and closer together.

When you start having contractions, let your health care provider know. Ask when you should go to the hospital. If you live nearby, this will likely be when you have contractions less than 5 minutes apart. The contractions should be strong and painful. If it takes a long time to get to the hospital, you might need to go sooner.

During early labor, your amniotic sac (bag of waters) may break. This is the sac of fluid in which your baby has been floating. When it breaks, you may feel a gush or trickle of warm fluid. Some of it may drip down your leg. Your water may break before or after contractions start. If it does, call your health care provider. You may be told to go to the hospital.

For several hours of your early labor, you may be at home. The hospital won't want to admit you until your contractions are close together and your cervix is dilating. They want to be sure you're truly in labor. Until then, comfort should be your goal. You and your labor helper can try the following:

- Walk around. This can help the contractions work better. Lean on your labor helper for support during contractions.
- Drink fluids and eat lightly. After labor starts, don't eat any big meals. Keep your body energized by drinking fruit juices and eating light foods.
- Take a warm bath to relax you. (If your water has broken, take a warm shower instead.)
- As each contraction starts, use breathing and relaxation exercises. Your labor helper can help you focus on these exercises. It will be important to rely on them as labor gets harder.
- Focus on a picture that makes you feel calm. Keep your arms and legs limp and let your uterus do the work.
- Change positions often to lessen discomfort. Any comfortable position is okay, except lying flat on your back. That position is not best for you or your baby.
- Rest. You and your labor helper will need your strength and energy for the big event ahead. Try to relax and get as much sleep as possible between contractions.

Once your contractions are very strong and come 10 minutes apart, you have entered a phase called active labor. Sometime during this phase you'll go to the hospital. In the hospital, your provider may decide a few procedures are needed. Some are routine, while others are used when problems are suspected. These procedures are explained in Figure 7-4. If your amniotic sac has not broken yet, your provider will decide the best time to break it.

As the cervix dilates to 8 or 9 centimeters, you enter the phase of labor called transition. This is the most difficult part of labor. Contractions will be very strong and painful. Your cervix is opening to 10 cm. You'll be working very hard, so try to rest between contractions. They will come about every 2 minutes and last about 45 to 90 seconds.

Medical Procedures Used in Childbirth

Labor	Delivery
Intravenous line (IV)—You can be given fluids or medicine through an IV if needed.	Forceps—a curved instrument that fits around the sides of the baby's head. Forceps are used to ease the baby down the birth canal while you're having a contraction.
Electronic fetal monitor—a wide belt that is placed around your abdomen and connected to a machine. The belt's sensor can detect the baby's heartbeat and measure your contractions. You may have this type of monitoring during pregnancy.	Vacuum extractor—a device with a soft rubber cup on the end. This cup fits around the top of the baby's head. The machine creates a vacuum suction that makes the cup hug the top of the baby's head. The provider can pull gently on it only during a contraction while you are pushing. This will ease the baby out of the birth canal.
Fetal scalp test—a blood test to see if the baby is getting enough oxygen. A very small blood sample is taken from the top of the head. It doesn't seem to hurt the baby. This blood can be quickly tested for oxygen content.	

7-4 Your health care provider should explain any procedures that will be done during labor and delivery. Don't be afraid to ask questions.

When your cervix is almost fully dilated, you may feel like vomiting. You may also feel shaky, hot and cold, and cranky. In this phase, you may be tired and frustrated. The calm words and gentle touch of a labor helper are important now. Your helper can also keep you focused on breathing and relaxation techniques. These are very helpful in this part of labor. You may feel the urge to push. <u>Do not push until your provider tells you to do so!</u>

The first stage of labor ends when your cervix is fully dilated to 10 cm. Soon labor will be over. It's a very intense experience. You may feel overwhelmed or be filled with many strong emotions. Remember this is a normal part of the process of childbirth.

Stage Two: Delivery of the Baby

The second stage of labor starts when your cervix is fully dilated. The purpose of this stage is to push your baby out of your uterus. See Figure 7-5. The length of stage two varies from woman to woman. The average time for pushing is about an hour for first pregnancies. In later pregnancies, stage two tends to be much shorter.

At this time, you will be told to push. You will use your muscles to push your baby out of the uterus. Pushing is done only during a contraction. These will be the strongest, longest contractions of all. Don't hold your breath during pushes—use your special breathing.

First, you will push the baby into the birth canal. It may feel like you're having a bowel movement. Don't be afraid of this feeling—it's normal. Next, you'll see the top of your baby's head at the opening of the birth canal. This is called crowning. It is an exciting moment!

When crowning occurs, your health care provider will decide if an episiotomy (ih-pee-zee-AH-tuh-mee) is needed. This is a small cut made at the opening of the birth canal to widen it. It gives your baby more room to be born. If you have an episiotomy, you may be given a local anesthetic to numb the area. This cut will be stitched after the baby is born.

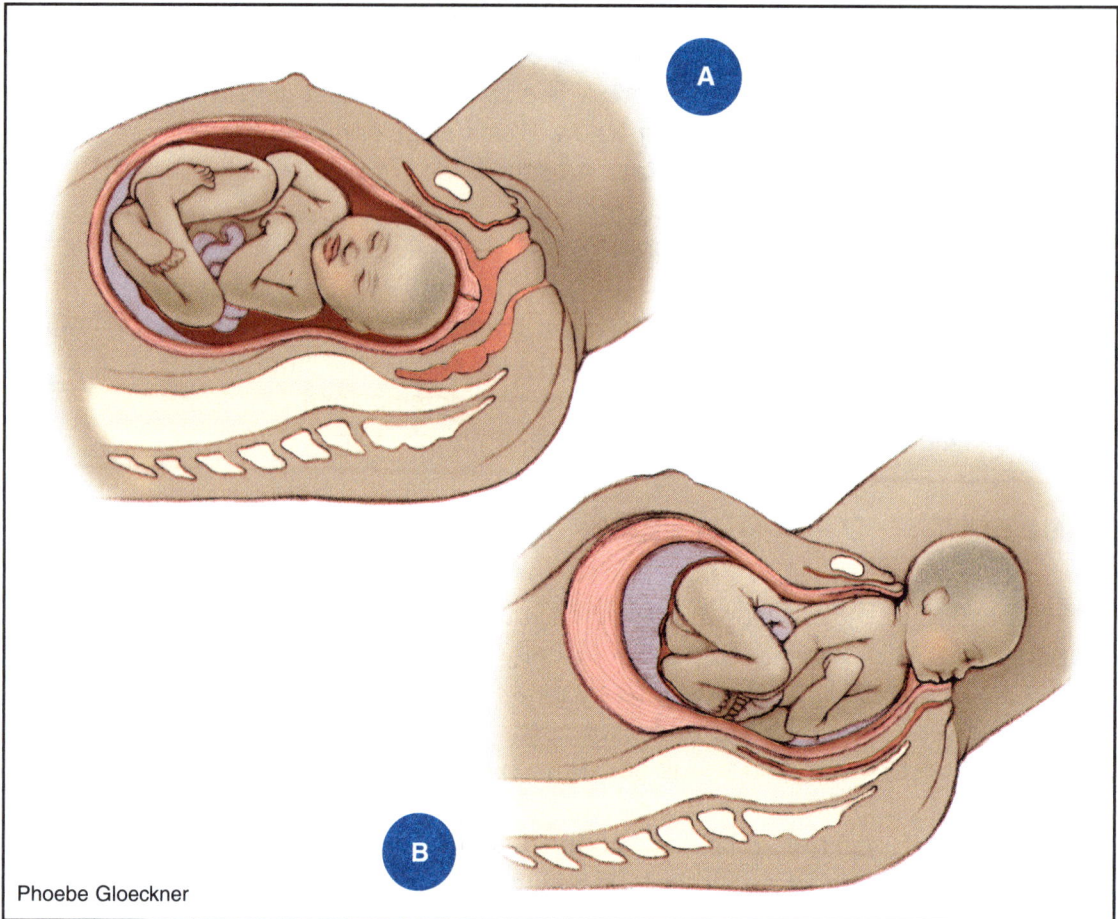

Phoebe Gloeckner

7-5 Before labor starts, the cervix is closed (A). As the second stage begins, the cervix is fully dilated and effaced (B). Now the mother can push her baby from her uterus.

When your baby's head is out, you'll feel less pressure on your vagina. The baby will turn her head to the side. This allows her shoulders to come out. Once the shoulders are out, the rest of her body will slide out quickly.

Soon you will hear your baby cry. Your baby's first cry is a sign her lungs are filling with air and she can breathe on her own. Your provider will hold the baby's head down to drain any mucus from her mouth and throat. A small suction bulb may be used to clear her airways. You may see specks of the white, waxy vernix on the baby's skin.

Your health care provider will clamp your baby's umbilical cord in two places. The cord will be cut between these clamps. Sometimes the baby's father or the labor helper can do this. If this is important to you, ask in advance whether this is an option at your hospital. Before the cord is cut, your baby will get oxygen from your blood through the placenta. Now the cord is no longer needed.

Stage Three: Delivery of the Afterbirth

The third stage of labor is the delivery of the afterbirth. This is the name for the placenta after the baby is born. Now the placenta is no longer needed. The body will expel it with a few contractions. It takes about 10 to 20 minutes for the afterbirth to pass from the uterus.

Your provider will check the placenta to make sure it is in one piece. None of it should be left inside you. That could cause you to bleed heavily. If you had an episiotomy, your provider will stitch the cut now. Your body will absorb these stitches in the weeks after pregnancy. You won't need to have them removed.

The nurse will massage your abdomen to make sure your uterus is contracting (getting smaller). This may hurt a little bit, but it's important. As the uterus contracts, this slows down the bleeding from your uterus. The nurse may show you how to massage your uterus, too.

After the delivery is over, you will be cleaned up and monitored very closely. The nurses will want to be sure you're recovering well. Your baby will be checked, too. In Chapter 8, you will read more about the medical care you and your baby will receive just after delivery.

Cesarean Delivery

The stages just described apply to vaginal births. Only about 70 percent of births in the U.S. are vaginal. The other 30 percent are cesarean deliveries. In a cesarean (sih-ZAIR-ee-uhn) delivery, an incision (cut) is made in the mother's abdomen and uterus. The baby is delivered through this cut. This operation can also be called a cesarean section or C-section.

This type of delivery is done when a vaginal birth is dangerous or impossible. It might occur for several reasons. Some C-sections are planned. The health care provider knows about a certain problem ahead of time. He or she tells the woman a cesarean delivery is needed. Then this surgery can be scheduled close to the due date. A C-section may be planned for the following reasons:

☞ The baby is in a breech position, which means he is head-up in the uterus. The head isn't against the cervix like it should be. Instead the baby is in a feet-first or sitting position. Sometimes the cervix doesn't open well when the baby is breech. Delivering a baby from this position can be dangerous. In this case, a cesarean will likely be done.

☞ The woman has had a prior cesarean delivery. It depends upon how the previous C-section was done. Most women who have had C-section can deliver vaginally in their next deliveries. This is called VBAC (vaginal birth after cesarean). Others may be advised to have another cesarean.

☞ The woman has a disease or infection the baby might get by entering the birth canal. This is most common with an STI, such as herpes or HIV. The woman's provider may choose cesarean delivery to protect the baby from coming into contact with the disease.

☞ The placenta is covering the cervix, blocking the baby from entering the birth canal (this is called placenta previa).

Cesarean deliveries are also used in emergencies. If vaginal delivery is not going as planned, the lives of both mother and baby can be at risk. See Figure 7-6 for reasons an emergency C-section may be needed.

You may wonder what to expect if you have a cesarean delivery. You'll be given medicine so you will not feel any pain. If you have an epidural, you will be awake but numb. With general anesthesia, you

Reasons for an Emergency Cesarean Delivery

❖ The baby's heart rate stays too low or the baby doesn't seem to be getting enough oxygen. This is described as fetal distress.

❖ Labor stops going as it should. This is called *failure to progress*. The cervix may not keep opening or the baby's head may be unable to come through the birth canal.

❖ Heavy and uncontrollable bleeding. This might occur as a result of problems with the placenta.

❖ Problems with the umbilical cord. The cord might wrap around the baby's neck or come through the birth canal first, cutting off the baby's oxygen supply.

7-6 Sometimes an emergency cesarean delivery is needed to protect the health of mother and baby.

would be asleep. A curtain will be placed across your stomach so you won't see what is happening. If you want your labor helper in the operating room with you, ask if this is okay. Some hospitals allow it, while others will not.

Your baby will be lifted out of your abdomen through the incision. If you are awake, you may feel this, but it won't hurt. Then you can hold or see your baby. If you're asleep, your labor helper may be able to hold him. Next your uterus and abdomen will be stitched. This will take about half an hour. Then you will be sent to a recovery room. Here, nurses will monitor you closely for a few hours.

After Delivery

Whether you deliver vaginally or by cesarean, you will be glad to finally see your baby. You have waited several months, and now you can meet her face to face! You will never forget this moment.

When the baby is given to you, you may want to put her directly on your chest. You can wrap the blanket around both of you. This way you can be skin-to-skin with your new little one. Your body and the blanket will keep her warm. Babies are usually very alert right after delivery.

Now is a good time to begin to get to know your newborn. Your baby has just made a dramatic transition to a new environment. She went from the coziness of your uterus to the outside world. She needs the comfort of your voice and the security of your body. Holding and talking to your baby is your first important task as a new mother.

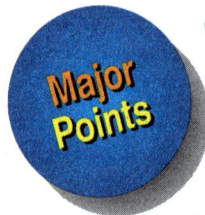

Major Points

☞ Childbirth is a process through which a baby is born. It involves labor and delivery.

☞ Physical changes during the last weeks of pregnancy mean your body is getting ready for labor and birth. Knowing what to expect can help you identify the start of labor.

☞ Before you go into labor, talk to your health care provider about your wishes regarding pain medication during childbirth. You can use breathing and relaxation exercises to cope with labor or ask for pain relief medication.

☞ Labor is divided into three stages. Each stage plays an important role in your baby's birth.

☞ A cesarean delivery may be needed if complications prevent a vaginal birth. This type of delivery may be planned or done on an emergency basis.

☞ Immediately after delivery, you and your new baby can start getting to know one another. Holding your baby close will comfort him or her after the stress of delivery.

Chapter 8
New Mom,
New Baby

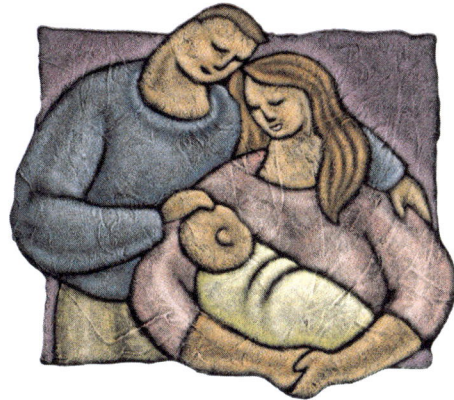

Immediately after delivery, you will feel a big relief. Your baby is finally here! You may also feel a bit overwhelmed. Having a baby is a very emotional experience. If you're making an adoption plan for your baby, you may have mixed feelings. If you plan to parent, you'll be happy to see and hold him. At the same time, you may not feel like you're a mother yet. You may cry and not know why. Your body is going through many changes, too. You may feel a little shaky and cold. It's been hard work and you're very tired.

This chapter tells what to expect in the days after childbirth. It explains changes you and your baby will experience in the postpartum period. Postpartum (pohst-AHR-tuhm) means right after childbirth. The first six weeks after delivery are known as the postpartum period. Some changes occur while you're still in the hospital. You will notice others after you return home.

While you're recovering, it's important to take care of yourself. Your body needs time to rest and mend itself from pregnancy and childbirth. If you're parenting, you can also use this time to get to know your new baby. This will be the beginning of parenthood, even if you don't feel like a parent just yet.

The Hours After Delivery

In the hours just after delivery, you and your baby will be recovering. Both of you will need certain medical care. The hospital staff will want to make sure both of you are in the best of health.

They will monitor you carefully and provide the care you need. In some cases, your baby may need special medical care. This would be given at this time.

If all goes well, you and your baby can start getting to know one another. Your labor helper may want to hold her, too. Your parents and the baby's father may not have been with you for the delivery. If not, they may want to see you and the baby now. This is an exciting time.

If you plan to breast-feed, put your baby to your breast right after delivery. This is important. Just after birth, she will be wide awake and ready to learn to breast-feed. It will be easier to get her to latch onto your breast and start to nurse. Nursing signals your brain to produce the hormones that make milk. It also tells your brain to make the hormones that contract your uterus. Contractions of the uterus help slow bleeding. If you need help with breast-feeding, ask a nurse to show you how. Keep asking until you have the help you need.

Medical Care of the Newborn

After birth, your baby's umbilical cord will be cut. His nose and mouth will be cleaned with a suction bulb. This will drain any mucus from his airways. The nurse will wipe him off with a warm, soft towel. He may be weighed and measured at this time. It's also possible this will happen later. An identification bracelet will be placed on his wrist or ankle. This matches your ID bracelet. To prevent bleeding and infection, your baby will be given a vitamin K shot and special eyedrops. He may be tested for anemia and other serious diseases.

Within a few minutes of birth, your baby will be given a brief exam. This is done to make sure he's healthy. The health care provider will check his color, breathing, heart rate, responsiveness, and muscle activity. The provider will rate him in each of these areas. As a result of this exam, your baby will receive a score that describes his condition. See Figure 8-1. This score is called an Apgar score. It's named after the doctor who created this

Apgar Score

Sign	Score 0	Score 1	Score 2
Heart Rate	Not beating	Beating slower than 100 beats a minute	More than 100 beats per minute
Breathing	Not breathing	Slow or irregular	Good; crying
Muscle Tone	Limp	Some movement	Active movement
Responsiveness	No response	Weak response	Alert; responsive
Skin Color	Blue	Body pink; limbs blue	Body and limbs pink

8-1 Dr. Virginia Apgar created this test to check an infant's condition at birth. After delivery, you can ask your provider about your newborn's Apgar score.

exam. A second Apgar score will be given about five minutes after the first. If your baby has an Apgar score of less than 7, he may need special medical attention.

Emergency Care

Most of the time, babies are born perfectly healthy. Sometimes, however, a newborn may need more than routine medical care. This might happen for a number of reasons. See Figure 8-2. No matter what the reason, this can be alarming for new parents. This is especially true if they didn't expect the baby to be ill. The joy of the baby's birth can be quickly overshadowed by fear of what will happen next.

When Is Emergency Care Needed?

* premature birth
* low-birthweight
* drug addiction
* very low Apgar score
* other serious health conditions

8-2 A newborn might need emergency medical care for any of these reasons.

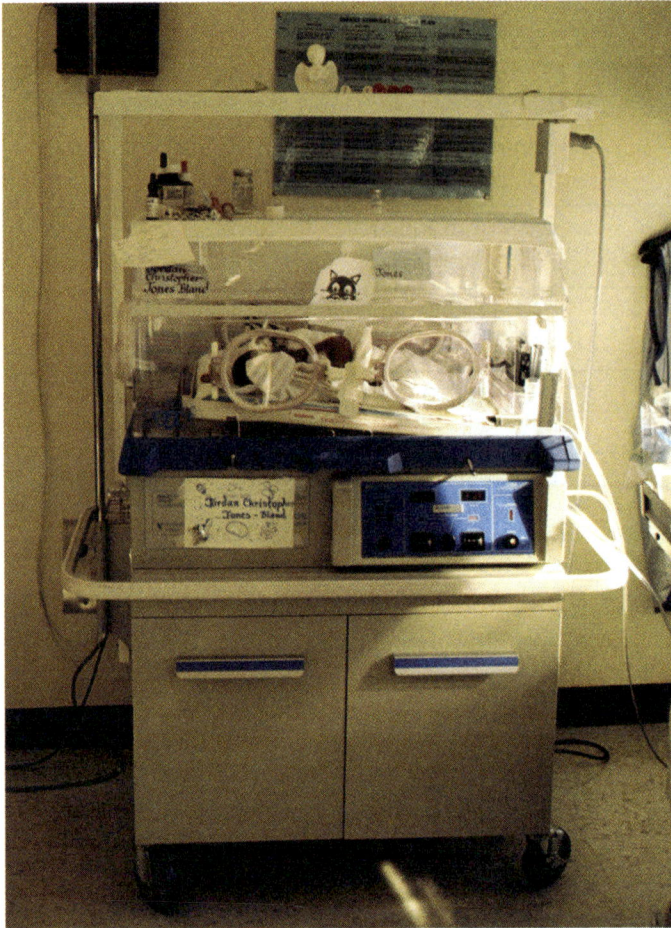

If your baby is ill, he might need to be placed in the newborn intensive care unit. Here he can receive the best care possible. He might need to be kept in an incubator. This special bed keeps your baby warm and reduces his exposure to germs. See Figure 8-3. He may be connected to machines by various tubes and wires. This can be a scary sight for new parents. It may help to remember the machines are working to help the baby until he is strong enough to come home.

If your baby needs emergency care, the best thing you can do is to stay calm. This can be difficult, but it's important. Ask your provider to explain the problem and what will be done about it. Your provider wants to give your baby the best possible care. He or she should also let you know what is happening to your baby. There are never any silly questions when it comes to your baby's health.

8-3 The incubator protects this fragile newborn. Through the holes in the sides, medical staff and the parents can touch and care for the baby.

Medical Care of the New Mom

For the first hour or so after delivery, the nurses will monitor your condition very closely. They will take your temperature, heart rate, and blood pressure every few minutes. Don't be alarmed—this is normal. The nurses just want to be sure your body is recovering well.

Right after delivery, you may feel hungry. No wonder! You've worked very hard and will need to eat. You may be very thirsty, too. In labor, you probably sweated a great deal. Drink lots of fluids. Major hormone and fluid changes are happening. These changes will cause you to urinate more often than usual.

You will notice a discharge from your vagina. This is called lochia (LOH-kee-uh). It is created by the pulling away of the placenta from the uterus. You will have lochia even if you had a cesarean delivery. At first, this discharge is bright red and may have some clots in it. You should not use tampons to absorb the lochia. Your cervix is still soft and open. Instead, use a sanitary pad. You will probably receive some extra large pads to use while you're in the hospital.

For the first 24 hours after childbirth, you may be given a cold pack to place on your sanitary pad. The coolness helps reduce swelling. After 24 hours, warm water on the area is recommended. This is especially true if you had an episiotomy or any small tear of the vagina. The nurses may give you a special basin called a sitz bath to sit in. The warm water can make the area feel better and heal faster. It also helps keep the area clean.

Your uterus will start to get smaller right away. Just after delivery, you'll be able to feel the top of it just below your belly button. The nurse will massage your abdomen and may show you how to do it, also. This stimulates the muscles of the uterus to contract. These contractions help slow the bleeding from your uterus.

With these contractions, you may feel some cramping. Some people call these cramps afterbirth pains. They are normal and will probably go away in a few days. If you're bothered by these cramps, ask your health care provider for some medication to relieve the pain.

If you had a cesarean delivery, it will take you longer to recover. You have just had major surgery and your body has to heal. Your hospital stay will be longer with this type of delivery. Your incision must heal. It will be closed with either stitches or metal staples. The stiches are usually absorbed by your body, but the metal staples must be removed.

While you're in the hospital, you may need pain medication. After a cesarean, you may also need help getting up. Getting out of bed and walking is good for you. Activity helps you avoid complications that can happen after any surgery. These include blood clots in your legs, lung infections, or a buildup of gas in your intestines.

Bonding Begins

Bonding describes the unique strong attachment that develops between parents and baby. When you hold and talk to your baby, she responds to you. You respond to her, too. The way the two of you interact makes you feel connected and close to each other. This natural process is bonding, and it can start right after birth. Fathers also bond with their babies when they hold and talk to them.

Bonding is critical for a healthy parent-child relationship. This attachment is necessary for both a mother and her newborn. It motivates a mother to be patient and provide all the care her newborn needs. For the newborn, being attached to at least one person (usually the mother) is critical for healthy development. Bonding builds a sense of basic trust about the world. This promotes healthy emotional growth.

Your baby's brain will continue to develop after birth. This development depends upon the stimulation she receives. You can help build your baby's brain by holding and talking to her! This is as important as feeding her. Babies who aren't talked to and held become withdrawn. They don't learn how to respond to or learn about the world.

Holding and talking to a newborn also communicates love. See Figure 8-4. Your baby can't understand the words you say, but the sound of your voice comforts her. She will become attached to you by being softly spoken to and gently held. Talk to your baby when you feed her, change her diaper, or bathe her.

Another way to communicate is to hold your baby in front of you with her eyes level with yours. Hold her six to nine inches from your face. Now talk softly to her. Keep talking while she tries to find and focus on your face. It will take a few minutes, but soon your baby will focus and find your eyes. Her eye muscles are still weak and uncoordinated. She may not be able to focus for very long, but she will enjoy this activity.

At times, you may not be able to get your baby to focus. This may happen when many people have been holding and talking to her. Babies can get overstimulated and need quiet. They may show this by a change in behavior or crying. Behavior changes you may see are avoiding eye contact, sneezing, hiccupping, spitting up, fussing, arching her back, or straightening her arms down the side of her body. Stop playing with your baby and ask other people to leave her alone for a while. Take your baby to a quiet area and hold her close. Talk or sing softly to her, but avoid making direct eye contact at this time. Provide gentle, repetitive motion for her, such as rocking, swaying, patting, or rubbing her.

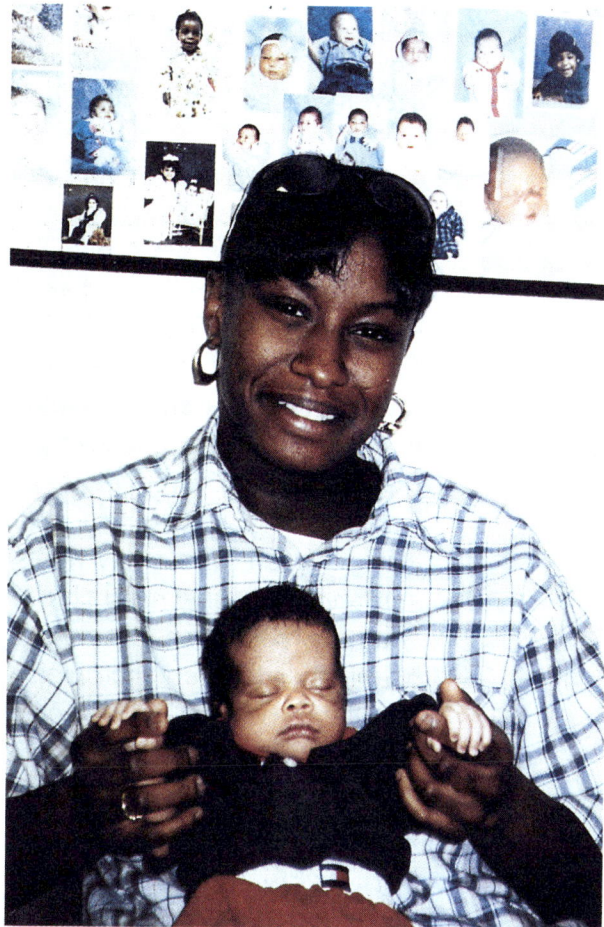

8-4 This mother strengthens her bond with her child when she holds him.

For a very young baby, you might also try swaddling. This means snugly but gently wrapping a thin blanket around your baby, but never over her face. Tuck her arms and legs inside the blanket against her body. This resembles the close quarters and warmth of the uterus. It can be soothing for very young babies. Before you leave the hospital, ask a nurse to show you how to fold the blanket to swaddle the baby. After about six weeks, though, many babies resist swaddling. Use other comfort measures for these older babies.

When your baby is overstimulated, she may need a few minutes by herself. She may want to just relax and stare off into space for a few minutes. Be sure she is in a safe place, such as her crib. Stay in the next room and check on her often. Never leave your baby alone in a house! She needs supervision even if you're not holding her.

By understanding your newborn's behavior, you will find it easier to bond with her. Keep in mind these behavior changes don't mean your baby is rejecting you. Often, they mean she needs a different type of attention. Don't take it personally. Instead, try something else to comfort her.

As a new parent, you will want friends and family to meet your new baby. It's a good idea to have most people wait until you have returned home from the hospital. You will be tired after childbirth. Feeding and caring for your baby will take much of your time and energy. If you have many visitors, you won't be able to rest much. You and your baby need this time alone to get to know one another. You may feel uncomfortable asking people not to come to the hospital or to keep their visits short. If so, ask a parent, nurse, or your labor helper to do it for you.

Early Decisions About Your Newborn

Before you leave the hospital, there are a few final decisions you need to make. If your baby is a boy, you'll need to decide about circumcision. You'll also need to make a final decision about the baby's birth certificate.

Circumcision

Circumcision (suhr-kuhm-SIH-zhun) is the removal of some of the loose foreskin that covers the male penis. Some parents choose to have this operation done on their male children. If you have a boy, you must decide whether to have him circumcised. This decision is best made before birth.

Some people favor circumcision. They believe it's healthier for the baby. Some studies show circumcision reduces the risk of urinary tract infections. Removing part of the foreskin can make it easier to clean the penis. Religious reasons may also play a role. In some faiths, it is required that baby boys be circumcised. Some people choose circumcision because it is tradition in their families. Studies are examining if a circumcised male has less risk of HIV.

Not all parents choose circumcision. Some see no need for it. The decision is yours. You can discuss circumcision with your family, the baby's father, your health care provider, or a pediatrician. Their opinions can help you decide. If you want your son circumcised, it is best to have this done before he leaves the hospital. If you have your son circumcised, ask his health care provider how to care for the area until it heals. This usually takes only a few days.

Baby's Birth Certificate

The baby's birth certificate is the legal document that proves she was born. She will need this important document all her life. On the birth certificate, you will provide your baby's legal name. By this time, you should have chosen her name. You may have a choice whether to give her your last name or her father's last name. This depends upon the laws of your state.

As the baby's mother, you will sign the birth certificate. Be sure all the information listed is correct. If anything is wrong, have the hospital correct it before you sign. Make sure your baby's name is spelled correctly. Otherwise, the incorrect spelling will be her legal name. Then, you would have to go to court to have it changed.

If the baby's father is present, have him sign the birth certificate, too. In some states, you can't list him as the father on the birth certificate unless he signs. In many states, his signature is a legal sign he claims the baby as his. If you have any questions about the father and the birth certificate, you may want to seek legal advice before the baby is born.

In most states, the hospital sends birth certificate information to the state's birth registry. You can get the official birth certificate in a few weeks. Ask the hospital what you need to do to get a copy. This might include paying a fee and going to the courthouse.

You may need proof of your baby's birth for welfare or Medicaid. Most hospitals can give you a statement to take home. Others provide an unofficial copy of the birth certificate for the parents. The baby's fingerprints or footprints may be on this copy.

Going Home from the Hospital

In the first few days after your baby is born, much is happening. Your body is recovering, and you are learning to care for your little one. Your hospital stay will end soon. Then you will be back at home. After a vaginal delivery, you will likely stay in the hospital less than two days. With a cesarean delivery, the stay is usually not more than four days.

You may not feel ready to leave the hospital. It might seem too soon. You might be anxious because you think you don't know all you'll need to know. Almost every new parent feels this way. You will quickly learn to care for your baby and meet his needs. To help new mothers, many hospitals arrange to have a nurse visit them at home soon after discharge. Other hospitals may have a nurse call you at home. Either way, the nurse would want to make sure you and the baby are doing well. See Figure 8-5.

Caring for Yourself

New mothers experience many dramatic physical and emotional changes. The physical changes may make you wonder if you'll ever feel good about your body again. You may be surprised by emotional and mood changes. Above all, it is important to take care of yourself. Accept help from those close to you at this time. Care and nurturance from others can help you adjust to being a new mother.

Physical Changes

Your body was changing over several months while you were pregnant. Now it will take some time for your body to get back to normal. For instance, it takes about two weeks for the uterus to return to its normal size. Allow six weeks to be sure the cervix is closed again.

During this time, it is important to refrain from sexual intercourse. Your cervix and vagina need time to recover. If you have stitches, these need to stay in place until the episiotomy or tear heals. Having sex too soon may cause them to come loose. Your body is also more vulnerable to infection at this time. Finally, having intercourse before you're fully healed can be quite uncomfortable. Ask your health care provider how long you should wait. During this time, show your affection for your partner in other ways. You might be too tired to even think about sex right now anyway.

You will continue to have lochia for as long as six weeks after delivery. This bright red discharge will change to a lighter pink or brownish color after a few days. Then, it will become thinner and almost

8-5 This nurse is preparing for a home visit with a new mother and her baby. Ask if your hospital has nurses who do home visits with new moms.

white or clear in color. Lochia has a unique scent, but it should not smell bad. If it does, you may have an infection. Tell your health care provider about this.

Your episiotomy or stitches may still bother you for a few days after you return home. Continue to use a sitz bath or soak in the tub at least once a day. This can make you more comfortable and help you heal faster. Your body will absorb the stitches in about two weeks. They do not have to be removed.

In the first days after childbirth, changes in your breasts might cause you some discomfort. Whether you breast-feed or not, you may have some initial swelling. Wear a comfortable bra day and night. Rest assured these changes won't last long.

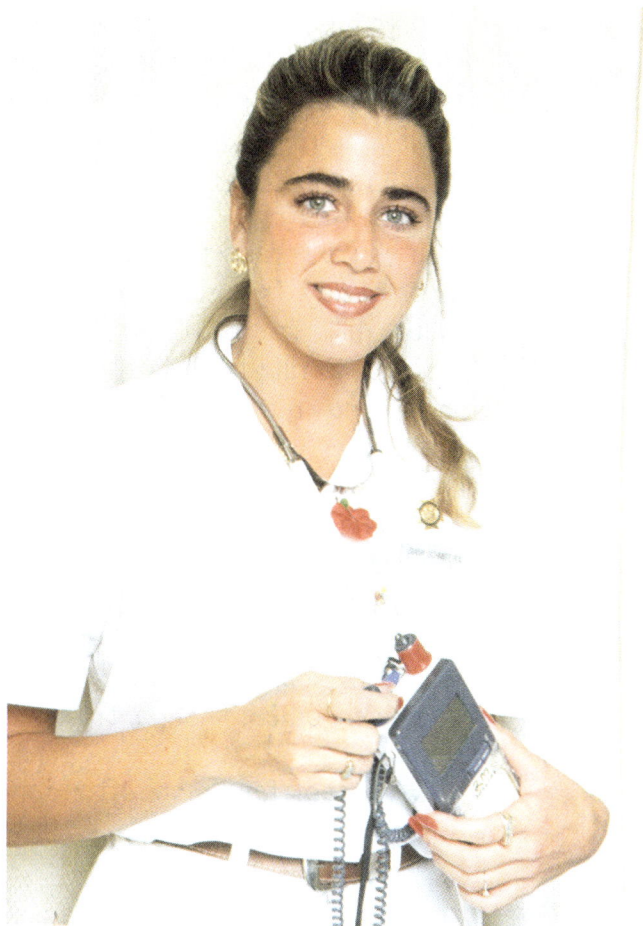

If you aren't breast-feeding, your breasts will naturally stop producing milk. No medication is needed to "dry up" the milk. You may have some tenderness for a few days. Cold compresses can help if you are uncomfortable. <u>Do not empty the breasts—this only causes them to make more milk!</u>

If you're breast-feeding, you will have increased swelling about the third day. This is a sign your breasts are starting to make mature milk. This swelling can be a little uncomfortable, but it won't last long. During this time, focus on the benefits of breast-feeding for you and your baby. This will help you keep the situation in perspective.

When your milk comes in, the worst thing you can do is breast-feed less. This might lead to engorgement (ihn-GORJ-muhnt), a painful condition in which the breasts become swollen, hard, and sore. It means the breasts are making more milk than is being used. By nursing your baby often, you can prevent engorgement. If you do become engorged, though, try the following:

- Breast-feed more often for about 24 hours.
- Place a warm, moist towel over your breasts or take a warm shower.
- Express a little milk to make you more comfortable. You can do this with your hands or a breast pump.

These measures should reduce your discomfort. In a day or so, your body will adjust. It will make only as much milk as your baby needs. Then your breasts will not be sore.

If just one spot on your breast is sore, you may have a clogged milk duct. This doesn't happen to every woman, but it can happen if the baby doesn't drain all the milk from your breast. Place a warm towel on it and then massage it. That may be enough to unclog the duct. If not, breast-feed a little more. If you have a fever or the sore spot gets red, call your health care provider. You may have mastitis. Mastitis (mas-STY-tuhs) is an infection of a milk duct in the breast. It may happen when milk stays in a milk duct and becomes infected. Your health care provider may prescribe antibiotics to treat this.

Another concern new moms have is getting their figures back. You may wonder how long it will be before you can fit into your regular clothes again. You will lose about 12 to 15 pounds within a few days after delivery. Some of it will be fluid. Six weeks later, you may have lost another 10 to 15 pounds.

The initial weight loss may not make as big a difference in how your clothes fit as you thought it would. Your muscles were stretched for many months and have lost some of their tone. Exercise will help you restore tone to your muscles. Speak to your health care provider about when to begin exercising. You can start with exercises you did during pregnancy. Eating nutritious foods can help you maintain your strength. Do the best you can. You may not have much appetite in the first weeks at home.

New moms also need plenty of rest. Rest gives your body time to repair itself. It helps you stay healthy. Getting enough rest in the first few weeks with a new baby is challenging. Ask others to help you complete tasks so you can rest. Sleep when the baby sleeps.

Emotional Changes

Physical changes aren't the only changes you may notice after childbirth. New mothers often have many emotional ups and downs. Your moods may go back and forth. Most of the time you can't explain the mood changes.

They are partly related to hormone changes that happen after childbirth. Other changes may contribute to the mood swings. You have been anxious to have your baby. Now that she is here, you may feel suddenly overwhelmed. When you were pregnant, especially in the last few months, you were the focus of much attention. Now most of the attention is on her.

You may have more sad than happy feelings for a while. You may feel down or cry for no reason. You may be grouchy or think no one cares about you. These feelings are so common after childbirth that people call them the baby blues. It can take a few days or even weeks for your moods to return to normal. If you have the baby blues, try the tips on the following page.

☞ Sleep when your baby sleeps. You are probably sleeping less now. Fatigue and exhaustion can make the blues worse. If you can, ask someone to care for your baby once in a while so you can have a longer period of sleep.

☞ Do something for yourself. Take a walk, wash your hair, put on makeup, or talk to a friend. Have someone watch your baby so you can have some personal time. See Figure 8-6.

☞ Make time for some exercise every day. Exercising will brighten your moods a little. Start slowly and gradually do more.

Keep in mind it is normal to feel disorganized and somewhat isolated for the first few weeks. Things will get better. Your body will return to normal. Your baby will sleep longer at night after a few weeks. You will start to enjoy being a new mother.

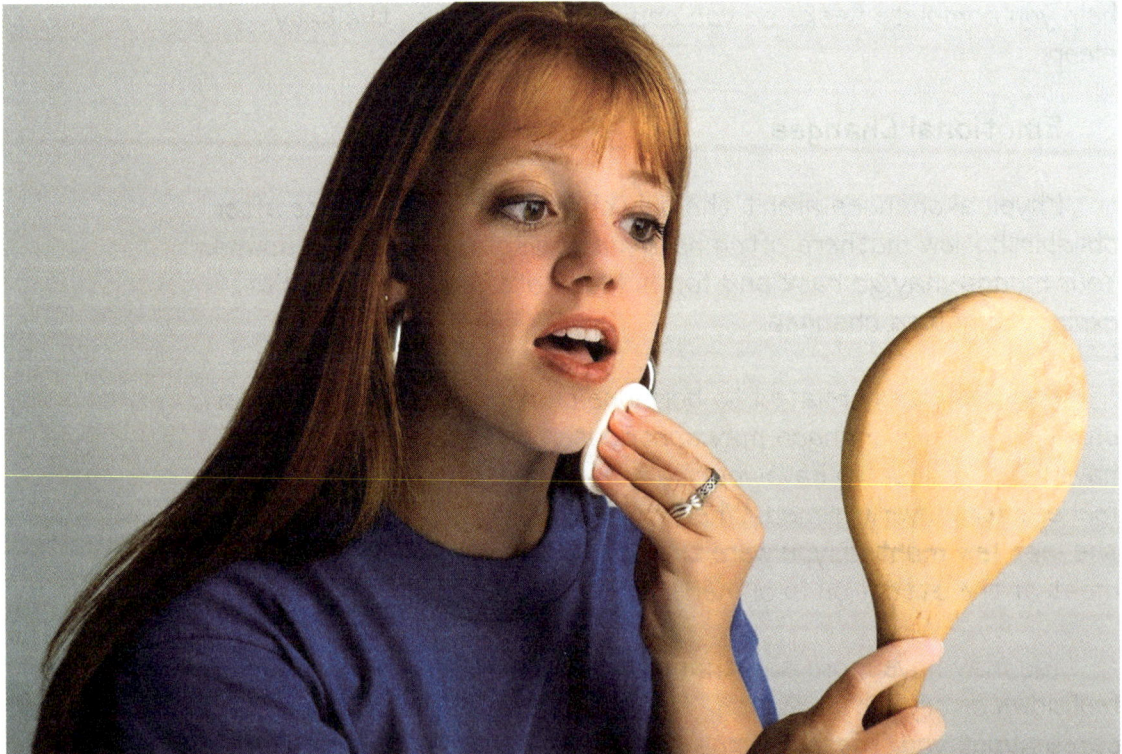

8-6 Taking a few minutes to do something you enjoy is a good way to manage stress. Putting on some makeup makes this teen feel her best.

Some women develop a serious depression after childbirth. It is called postpartum depression. It is not common and needs medical treatment. Symptoms include the following:

- ☛ unable to stop crying
- ☛ changes in the amount of sleep (much more or less than usual)
- ☛ feeling unable to take care of yourself
- ☛ feeling unable to take care of your baby

If you have any of these feelings, talk about them with someone you trust. Let your health care provider know. Talking to a counselor may help. It is important to resolve postpartum depression right away. Otherwise, you won't be able to care for yourself and your child as you should.

If you made an adoption plan for your baby, you probably have mixed feelings. You may wonder if you did the right thing. What you did takes a lot of emotional strength. It's hard to do what you think is best for your baby when it makes you feel so bad. You may miss her and grieve because she's not with you. You may feel relieved and guilty at the same time. Talking with someone about these feelings is very important. Most adoption agencies arrange for follow-up counseling for birthmothers. Your health care provider can also help you find counseling.

Postpartum Checkup

You will need a medical checkup about six weeks after childbirth. At this checkup, your health care provider wants to make sure your body is returning to normal. He or she will examine your breasts, uterus, cervix, and vagina. Your blood pressure and weight will be checked. A blood test may be done if you had anemia during pregnancy. At this visit, you can talk to your provider about any concerns you may have. Many teen moms ask about nutrition, exercise, and weight loss.

Instead of a six-week checkup, you might have an appointment two to four weeks postpartum. Your health care provider may want to talk to you about being a new mom, breast-feeding, returning to school, and birth control.

If you had a cesarean delivery, you may also need an appointment sooner than six weeks. Your provider may need to check your incision. If so, you may have a second checkup six weeks after delivery.

Birth Control

Right now, being pregnant again may be the last thing on your mind. However, it's very important not to become pregnant again before you're ready. Most teen parents say they don't want another baby for a few years. Most likely, you will want to postpone another pregnancy, too. Your next baby will be healthier if you avoid pregnancy for at least two years.

Your ability to become pregnant returns within a couple of weeks after delivery. Think ahead and form a plan. Talk to your health care provider and your partner. If you have a plan in place, you'll be more likely to successfully postpone pregnancy.

Many teens choose abstinence (postponing sex) after childbirth. They know it's the only guaranteed way to prevent pregnancy. For this method to work, you and your partner must agree about postponing sex. The two of you must decide what you will do that will help you abstain from sex. The success of this method depends on self-control—yours and your partner's. The benefits make this option worth it, though. You and your partner can talk about how to postpone sex until you are ready. By working together, you and your partner can make your relationship stronger.

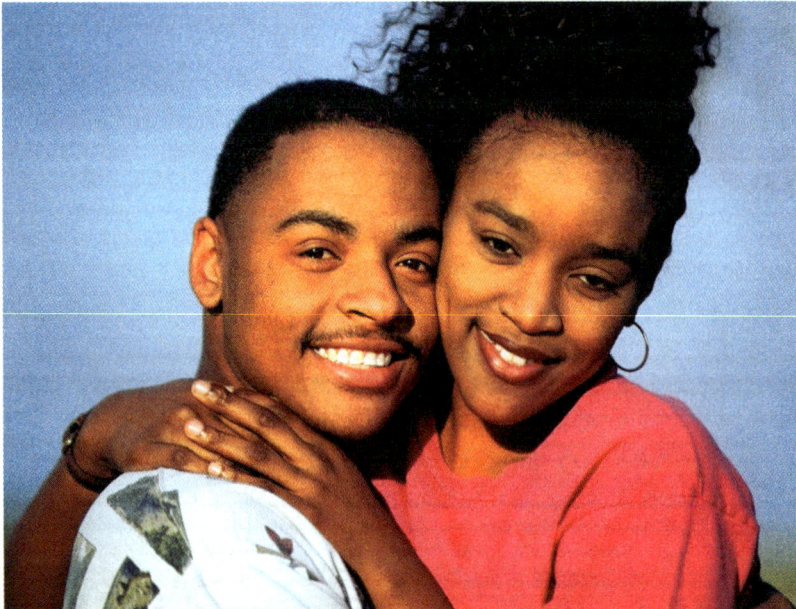

8-7 Couples can show their love in other ways than by having sex. Waiting allows a couple to focus on their relationship.

Even if you choose abstinence, you should learn what methods of birth control are available. Ask your health care provider about your options.

If you're breast-feeding, you may be able to take a version of the birth control pill called the minipill. This pill does not contain estrogen and is considered safe for the baby. It also seems to help milk production. It is also considered safe to start hormone injections or hormone implants six weeks after birth. Breast-feeding does not protect you from pregnancy. This is a myth.

If you're bottle-feeding, most forms of birth control can be started right away. For instance, you can receive a hormone injection before you leave the hospital. Birth control pills may be started soon after your baby is born.

You could also choose a birth control method that does not rely on the use of hormones. These methods can be started right away. Your health care provider can help you choose the method that's right for you. (See another title in this series, Understanding Your Changing Life, for more about birth control.)

Your Newborn's Abilities

Getting to know your baby is a very important task. It takes time. Plan to spend lots of time with your baby for the first few weeks. As you watch him, you will learn his signals. It will become easier for you to know what he needs. With each passing day, you will feel more confident as a mother.

You may wonder what your newborn can do. Newborns are small and helpless, but they are born with certain abilities that help them learn and grow. Your baby can't do many of the things he will do when he is older. But when you consider that he was just born, some of his abilities may surprise you!

Hearing

Your newborn can hear very well. In fact, her sense of hearing started to work when she was still inside your uterus. Some studies have shown newborns can be calmed by listening to soothing music their mothers played often during pregnancy. Soft, familiar sounds are comforting. Your baby will also recognize your voice. Soon after birth, she will respond to your voice by turning her head toward it.

Hearing is one of the first ways a newborn learns about the world. Through hearing, she begins to get to know you. Her brain development also is stimulated as she hears sounds and learns to connect them with people or events.

Sucking

Another ability of newborns is sucking. Babies can suck and swallow in the uterus before birth. By the time he is born, your baby can do this very well. Sucking is vital to survival, because this is how he eats. Sucking can also be comforting. This explains why babies may need to suck on their fingers, fists, or pacifiers. See Figure 8-8.

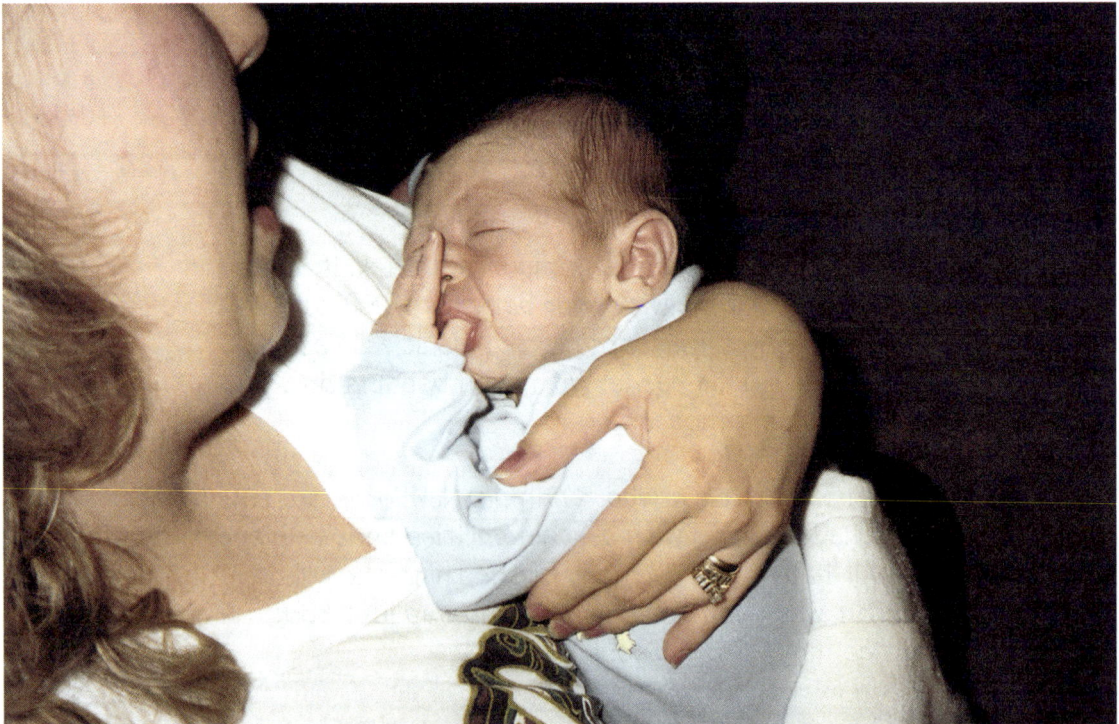

Bonnie Mori

8-8 This newborn sucks on his fingers for comfort. This relaxes him.

Crying

Your newborn has only one way to communicate—crying. She doesn't cry because she wants to. She cries because it's her only way to tell you she feels uncomfortable. Soon, you may be able to tell what your baby needs by the way she cries. For instance, a hunger cry may differ from her pain cry.

At times you may try everything to comfort her with no success. This usually means she just needs to be held or comforted. Hold your baby when you hear this cry. When you respond to her needs, she'll develop a sense of trust. This trust promotes healthy emotional growth.

It can be hard to listen to so much crying. Remembering the limits of your newborn's abilities may help. She is not capable of wanting to do something. Her brain is not developed enough to think and then act. She is not being evil, greedy, or intentionally demanding. She can only respond to her feelings of pain, comfort, hunger, discomfort, and sleepiness by crying.

Smelling

Every person has his or her own body scent. This natural scent is not from any perfume or cologne. At birth, your baby has a pretty good sense of smell. When you hold him, he will quickly recognize your unique scent. In this way, he knows the difference between you and other people. Your baby may also respond to very strong odors with facial expressions or by crying.

Seeing

Your newborn's sight is not very well developed. She can see right after birth, but not clearly. Your baby will respond best to bright colors and sharp contrasts. For instance, she may like a pattern or large, bold, black-and-white stripes. Newborns also prefer to look at human faces.

The muscles in your baby's eyes are still weak and uncoordinated. This can make her eyes look crossed. This is normal and will go away as her muscles strengthen. If you're concerned about it, talk about it with your health care provider.

Your newborn can focus on your face when she is close to you, but it takes time. In fact, a newborn can see clearly only for a distance of 8 to 12 inches. Hearing your voice tells your baby where to focus her eyes. As she grows, she will be able to focus better for longer periods of time. Over time, she'll begin to see more clearly and farther away.

Touching

The sense of touch is well developed in a newborn. Your baby's skin is very sensitive to being touched. He notices temperature differences, too. Warmth and closeness mimic the sensation of being inside the uterus. This can make him feel secure. This sense of security promotes a sense of trust.

Your newborn cannot touch an object on purpose. If you place an object in his hand, he will instinctively grab it. Newborns can have a surprisingly strong grip! Your baby's brain cannot interpret what he touches, though. This will develop in time.

Your Newborn's First Checkup

If your baby was born at 37 weeks or later, she will need her first medical checkup about two weeks after birth. Babies born earlier than 37 weeks may need earlier and more frequent checkups. At the first checkup, she will be weighed and measured. The health care provider will check her carefully. Her eyes and ears will be examined. The provider will run any medical tests your baby needs. This is also a time for you to ask any questions about her eating, sleeping, and growth.

It is best to make this first appointment before you leave the hospital. Adjusting to a new baby will keep you busy. It will be easy to forget to make the appointment.

If you haven't found a health care provider for your baby, you should do so now. Using a nearby health facility can be convenient. Your baby will need frequent checkups. These visits can prevent serious illnesses and make sure she is growing well. It's easier to use a provider you can get to on your own. Depending on other people to take you to appointments can be stressful.

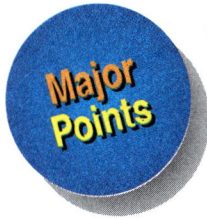

Major Points

☛ In the postpartum period, you will experience many physical and emotional changes. Your body will be recovering from childbirth and adjusting to not being pregnant anymore. Your newborn will be adjusting to life outside your uterus.

☛ In the hours after delivery, both the mother and baby need routine medical care. Throughout your hospital stay, the medical staff will provide this care. In some cases, emergency care may be needed.

☛ Bonding can begin just after birth. You and your baby can start growing attached to one another right away. This attachment is good for your parent-child relationship and the baby's emotional health.

☛ Before you leave the hospital, you have a few decisions to make. If you have a boy, one decision is about circumcision. Final information will also need to be given for the baby's birth certificate.

☛ Your recovery and adjustment don't end when you leave the hospital. You will continue to face changes even after you return home. During this time, it is important to take care of yourself.

☛ Your ability to become pregnant returns within two to three weeks after childbirth. Have a plan in place for preventing another pregnancy until you are ready.

☛ You need to have a postpartum checkup about six weeks after childbirth. This is done to be sure your body has healed from pregnancy and childbirth.

☛ Getting to know your baby is also important now. Babies are born with certain abilities that help them learn and grow. By observing your baby, you can learn what he can do.

☛ Your newborn will need a medical checkup soon after birth. At this visit, the health care provider will check the baby carefully to make sure she is healthy and growing properly.

Chapter 9
Caring for
Your Newborn

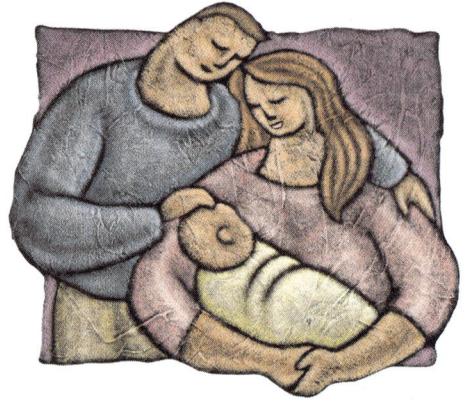

Your new baby will need a lot of care. At first, you may feel overwhelmed. This tiny, helpless creature depends on you to give him everything he needs. At times you may not even know <u>what</u> he needs. There's so much to learn.

Don't get discouraged, though. Soon you will be more comfortable handling your baby. With practice, you'll discover the best ways of feeding, diapering, and bathing him. In time, these routine care skills will seem like second nature. You'll learn how to plan what needs to be done. This chapter will explain newborn care. It will help you prepare to take care of your baby.

Medical Care

Your baby should have her first medical checkup soon after birth. This is the first of several routine checkups she will have. At these checkups, babies must get immunizations (ih-myuh-neh-ZAY-shunz) to prevent serious diseases. The baby's health care provider will tell you when these shots are needed. See 9-1 for a suggested immunization schedule for the first year. The provider will give you a small immunization booklet. Here you can record every shot your baby has. This is a very important record. Keep it up-to-date and store it in a safe place. Your child will need a current immunization record to enter a child care center or school.

You will have lots of questions about your baby. If you think of these between visits, write them down. You can take them with you to the baby's medical appointment. Every question is important. When in doubt about something, ask. Being involved in your baby's medical care will help you feel more confident in your role as a new parent.

Immunization Schedule—Birth to 18 Months

Immunization	When
Hepatitis B	Twice before 4 months 6 to 18 months
Diptheria, tetanus, and pertussis (DTaP vaccine)	2 months 4 months 6 months 15 to 18 months
Polio (inactivated polio vaccine-IPV)	2 months 4 months 6 to 18 months
Haemophilus influenzae Type b (Hib vaccine)	2 months 4 months 6 months 12 to 15 months
Measles, mumps, and rubella (MMR vaccine)	12 to 15 months
Chicken pox (varicella vaccine)	12 to 18 months
Rotavirus	2 months 4 months 6 months
Pneumoccal	2 months 4 months 6 months 12 to 18 months

9-1 The American Academy of Pediatrics recommends these immunizations in the first year and a half. Your baby's health care provider's recommendations may vary somewhat.

Feeding Your Baby

One of the first things you will do as a new mother is feed your baby. By the time your baby is born, you have probably decided how you will feed him. Many new mothers like breast-feeding. They enjoy the special closeness it gives them with their babies. If you try breast-feeding and don't like it, you can always switch to formula-feeding from a bottle. It's fairly easy to change from breast-feeding to bottle-feeding. Changing from bottle to breast is not so easy. Unless the baby nurses, your milk production will decrease drastically. Your milk will soon dry up and breast-feeding will no longer be an option.

Feeding your newborn is an important job that starts right after birth. No matter which method you use, there are a few key points to know. Most of these relate to your baby's health and safety. The following sections describe how to use each feeding method.

Breast-Feeding

If you've chosen to breast-feed, you may have a few questions about this method. You may even feel a little nervous. Learning to breast-feed takes time and patience. Once you and your baby are used to it, however, you will likely find this method is easy to use.

Breast Milk

Your body creates breast milk to nourish your baby. What is amazing is that your breasts adjust and change your milk to meet your baby's needs. The first milk your breasts make is called colostrum. It is a thick, clear, yellow fluid. Colostrum contains exactly what your baby needs in her first few days of life. It is rich in nutrients and easy to swallow. Colostrum also has a large number of antibodies in it. These antibodies help your baby fight disease. This is why nursing your baby is beneficial.

Transitional milk comes in about three days after birth. It lasts for two to three weeks. This milk is a mixture of colostrum and mature milk. (Mature milk is the milk your body will produce when breast-feeding is well established.) The ratio of colostrum to mature milk in transitional milk constantly changes. Over time, transitional milk will contain less and less colostrum.

By about three weeks after birth, your breasts will produce only mature milk. This milk is thin and white with a bluish tint. You may think the change in your milk means the milk is getting weak, but this is not true. This appearance is normal for breast milk. Mature milk is full of the nutrients your baby needs to grow and thrive. It will keep your baby healthy.

Breast-Feeding Techniques

When you are ready to breast-feed, begin by washing your hands. This helps reduce your baby's exposure to infections.

The most vital point about breast-feeding is the hold the baby's mouth has on your breast. This is called the latch-on. For a good latch-on, the baby's mouth must take in not only the nipple, but much of the areola (the darker part around the nipple). See Figure 9-2.

The baby's sucking action squeezes milk out of the ducts in the areola. When the baby has only the nipple in her mouth, not much milk comes out. She tries to get milk by sucking harder. Then you get sore nipples. You can tell when the baby is latched on well by looking for the following:

- Most of the areola is in the baby's mouth.
- Her lips are turned out against your breast, especially the bottom lip.
- Her nose is close to or pressing against your breast.

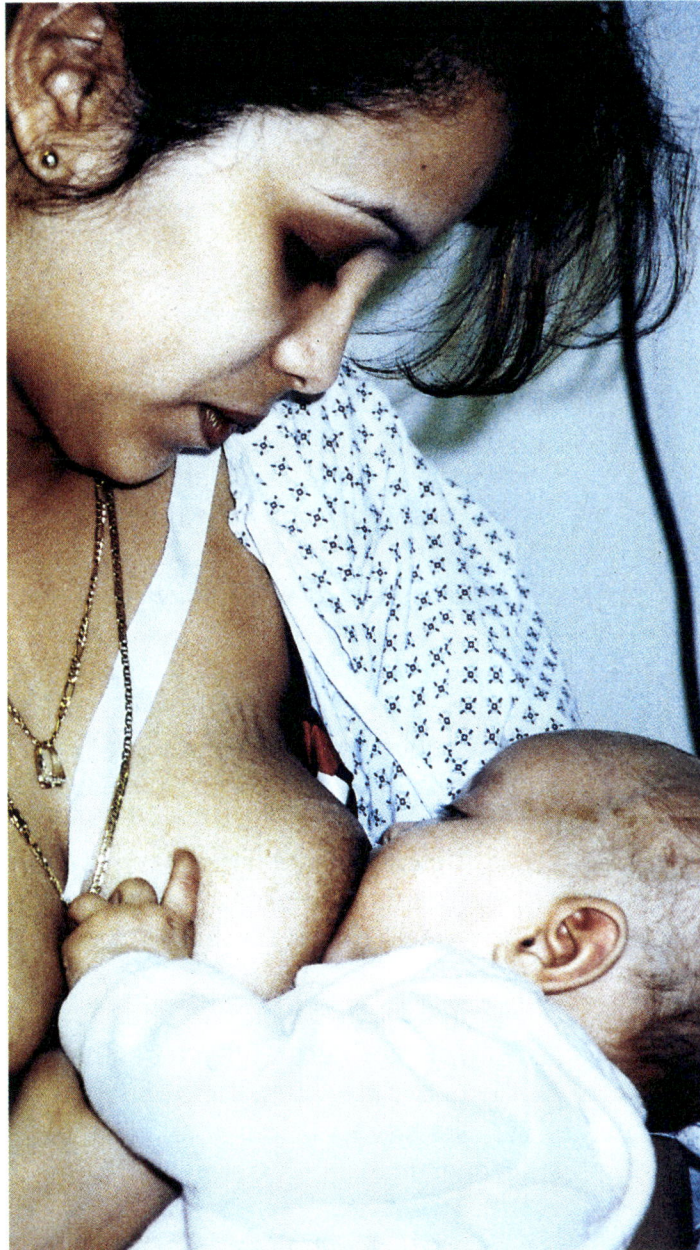

9-2 A correct latch-on is important. It allows baby to get milk from the breast without hurting the mother.

Usually, a good latch-on doesn't just happen. You have to make the baby's mouth open wide. To do this, hold your breast with your thumb on top near the outer edge of the areola. Place your other fingers underneath your breast. Gently move your nipple back and forth across your baby's lips. Soon her mouth will open wider. Quickly bring your baby to your breast. Hold her tummy-to-tummy so she faces your breast. Use your finger to lightly press your breast, giving her breathing room.

Use pillows or a folded blanket to support her during feedings. This makes it easier to keep your baby high enough to face your breast. It also keeps your arms from getting tired and your back from hurting.

Opinions differ as to how long the baby should nurse at each breast. Many mothers are advised to let the baby nurse 5 minutes on each breast at each feeding the first day. They can increase the time to 10 minutes on each side the second day. After the second day, allow your baby to nurse 15 minutes on one side and as long as she wants on the other side. During the first few weeks, it is important to let your baby build your milk supply to meet her needs.

To empty the breasts equally, begin the next 15-minute feeding on the side you finished with last. Let your baby nurse as long as she wants on the second side. Put a safety pin on your bra strap to remind you which breast to start with at the next feeding.

Be careful if you must remove the baby from the breast. Gently insert a finger into the baby's mouth to break the suction. Never try to pull the baby off your breast. This can cause sore nipples.

You may wonder if you have enough milk. Listen carefully to your baby as she nurses. If you can hear swallowing, she is getting milk. Also note how many times baby's diapers are wet each day. As long as she has six or more wet diapers every day, your baby is getting enough milk.

Most newborns breast-feed every 1½ to 2 hours. The time between feedings gradually increases to 3 or 4 hours. Don't be alarmed if some days your baby wants to nurse more than others. Your baby will go through several growth spurts. During this time, she will want to eat much more often. The first growth spurt usually occurs at two weeks. If you breast-feed frequently, your supply will increase within 24 hours to meet her needs. Fortunately, these growth spurts last only a couple of days.

Breast Pumps

You might consider using a breast pump to express (squeeze out) milk from your breasts. Then your baby's father or someone else can feed her some of the time. This is also helpful when you return to school. During the day, your baby's caregiver can bottle-feed your expressed breast milk to the baby. This is healthier for your baby than infant formula. In the mornings, evenings, and weekends, you can still breast-feed. Using a breast pump can help you keep breast-feeding even if you can't nurse for every feeding.

Not every breast pump is efficient and easy to use. Pumps with plastic storage bottles are preferred. Glass bottles are not recommended for use with breast milk. Glass attracts and holds the healthy antibodies. This keeps your baby from getting some of the benefits of breast milk. Before buying a pump, talk to a lactation consultant or childbirth educator. You can also call your local La Leche League. Ask what kind of pump to use, as well as how to use and clean the pump. Find out about safely collecting and storing the breast milk.

If you will be pumping daily, choose a good, electric breast pump. This may cost more, but it will contribute to your breast-feeding success. A lower-quality pump may cost less, but it may not work well enough to keep your milk supply up. It may also be less comfortable and harder to to use.

You can rent a breast pump from a hospital, as well as some pharmacies and lactation consultants. You can buy a pump from these and other sources, too. If you are enrolled in the Special Supplemental Nutrition Program for Women, Infants, and Children (WIC), ask if you can receive a breast pump. Some WIC offices give high-quality breast pumps to mothers in the program.

If you pay to rent or buy a breast pump, it may seem expensive. Actually, though, a good breast pump will pay for itself in time. Think of the money you will save on formula. You will also be able to use a quality pump longer than a less expensive one. If you have a second baby, you might even be able to use the breast pump again.

Concerns with Breast-Feeding

Breast-feeding involves both you and your baby. You may have some special concerns about your role in breast-feeding. For instance, you may wonder how your nutritional needs change while you breast-feed. You may wonder about substances being passed to your baby in your milk. Nipple soreness or modesty concerns are also common.

Nutrition. Your baby will get all his nutrients and fluids from your breast milk. Therefore, it is important for you to eat nutritious foods. Extra fluids are important also. Drink at least eight 8-ounce glasses of water, milk, or juice daily. Drinking some fluid every time you nurse your baby is a good idea.

It takes energy to make breast milk, so your body will need extra calories. The recommended amount is 500 more calories daily than before you were pregnant. You will also need certain nutrients in greater amounts now. Ask your health care provider or a dietitian about nutrient needs during breast-feeding.

You may find some foods seem to bother your baby. Spicy foods, garlic, onions, cabbage, and chocolate may cause your baby some discomfort. Observe carefully to learn which if any foods bother her. If you identify a problem food, you can limit or avoid this food.

Dangerous Substances. Almost everything you eat or drink enters your breast milk. For this reason, avoid substances that could endanger your baby. Alcohol, tobacco, and illegal drugs can pass into breast milk. So can caffeine from coffee, teas, and soft drinks. Teas may also contain some herbs that are dangerous for your baby. While breast-feeding you should limit caffeine intake. Avoid herbal teas, alcohol, tobacco, and illegal drugs.

Check with your health care provider before taking any medicines. Any prescription or over-the-counter medicine you take can pass to the baby in your breast milk. Many medicines will not harm your baby, but others are quite dangerous.

Nipple Soreness. Some nipple soreness is common when you begin breast-feeding. This should go away after a couple of weeks if you have a good latch-on technique. Air-drying your nipples after each feeding helps, too. Do not use soap to wash your nipples. This could remove the natural oils that protect the nipple. See Figure 9-3 for more tips on preventing nipple soreness.

Caring for Sore Nipples

❖ Hold the baby in the different positions from one feeding to the next. Use pillows or folded blankets to support the baby during feedings. This makes it easier to keep the baby high enough to face your breast.

❖ During feedings, make sure your baby's mouth is around the nipple and covers at least ¼- to ½-inch of the areola.

❖ If you must remove the baby from the breast during a feeding, remember to break the suction by inserting a clean pinky finger into the corner of the baby's mouth. Don't pull the nipple out of the baby's mouth, as this can hurt your nipple.

❖ After each feeding, spread a little breast milk around your nipple and areola. Let it air dry. Avoid using waterproof pads in your bra. These keep air from circulating to your nipple. Moisture will collect and cause more soreness.

9-3   If your nipples are sore from breast-feeding, try some of these suggestions.

Modesty. Some mothers are concerned about modesty when breast-feeding. Breast-feeding when others are present or when you're away from home can be done discreetly, but it takes a little planning. A nursing bra and the right clothing will help you nurse your baby and stay covered. Choose a blouse or sweater that opens in front or lifts easily. Have a small blanket with you to drape over your shoulder and your baby to shield your breast. Practice at home so you learn how to do this easily. As you become more used to breast-feeding, you may be more comfortable with nursing in public.

Bottle-Feeding

You can use a bottle to feed your child breast milk or infant formula. You might wonder what equipment you will need and what techniques to use for bottle-feeding. If you are using an infant formula, there are some additional tips to keep in mind.

When using a bottle, remember your newborn should drink only breast milk or infant formula (and water, if your baby's health care provider recommends it). Cow's milk is not recommended for babies before one year of age. It cannot provide the nutrients your baby needs in the proper amounts. Cow's milk is also very hard for the baby to digest. It is likely to cause allergies in your baby.

Bottle-Feeding Equipment

To bottle-feed, you will need the following equipment:

- 4 bottles with nipple units, 4-ounce size
- 10 to 12 bottles with nipple units, 8-ounce size
- utensils for formula preparation, such as a large measuring pitcher, measuring cup, can opener, long-handled mixing spoon, and tongs
- brushes to clean bottles and nipples
- a sterilizer (or you can sterilize equipment by putting it in a pan of boiling water)

You may wonder whether to buy glass or plastic bottles. Glass bottles are breakable, but easy to clean. They aren't recommended for use with breast milk, though. Plastic bottles work very well. Bottles with disposable liners can minimize the amount of air the baby swallows. They collapse as he feeds. These cost more.

Orthodontic nipples are recommended. Their shape allows a more natural sucking motion. This shape is most like the breast. It makes switching between bottle and breast easier for the baby.

Sometimes you may need to adjust the size of the hole in the nipple. To check the nipple hole, turn the bottle upside down and shake it gently. If it is the right size, formula will come out in a little spray and then a few drops. If it is too big, formula will pour or spurt out. You may notice your baby chokes during feedings or has formula leaking out around his mouth. Boil the nipple in water for about 10 minutes. If this doesn't make the hole smaller, buy a new nipple.

If the nipple hole is too small, only a drop or two of milk will come out. Your baby may suck very hard, seem unhappy, and release the nipple. You can make the nipple hole bigger. Heat a large safety pin or needle in a flame and poke it through the nipple hole. This will enlarge the hole.

Bottle-Feeding Techniques

You and your baby can feel very close if you use a bottle to feed him. Hold your baby during feedings. This is a great time to talk to and cuddle him. Newborns can't understand your words, but they can feel your love. This kind of nurturance is vital to a baby's emotional health. Never prop the bottle—your baby needs your attention during feedings. Propping the bottle can also lead to choking.

Remember to wash your hands before each feeding. You may wonder whether to heat the baby's bottle before giving it to him. You can warm it if you want, but you don't need to. The formula doesn't need to be very cold, either. Watch your baby to learn whether he seems to prefer his bottle warm.

To warm your baby's bottle, put it in a pan of warm water or hold it under running warm water. Test the heated liquid by putting a few drops on the inside of your wrist before offering it to the baby. Never warm the bottle in a microwave oven! The liquid may heat unevenly in the microwave. The part you test may be only warm, but other parts may be very hot and burn your baby's mouth. The bottle might also explode in the microwave if it is heated too long.

To feed your baby, hold him in a semi-upright position in your arms. If he lies flat while drinking, it increases his chance of choking and ear infection. Tilt the bottle so formula always fills the nipple. This also reduces the amount of air baby swallows. Swallowed air can result in gas, vomiting, or discomfort. This would make your baby very uncomfortable.

Infant Formula

Your baby's health care provider will help you choose a formula for your baby. If you think your baby needs a different formula, speak to the baby's health care provider first. If you're enrolled in WIC, the program will give some of the formula you need. You'll be responsible for buying the rest. Formula is quite expensive. It is estimated that formula-feeding an infant costs almost $2,000 per year using formula powder, which is the least expensive.

For the first 12 to 24 hours, your baby may not drink more than half an ounce of formula at each feeding. See Figure 9-4. As long as he has six or more wet diapers a day, he is getting enough. Before you leave the hospital, ask your nurse how much formula to offer your baby.

Infant formula comes in three forms: powder, concentrate, and ready-to-use. Formula sold in powder form must be mixed with a set amount of water before use. Formula concentrate is a liquid, but it also must be mixed with water. Ready-to-use formula can be used as is. Read the formula's label carefully, and follow the directions exactly. It can be harmful for your baby's health if his formula is not mixed properly.

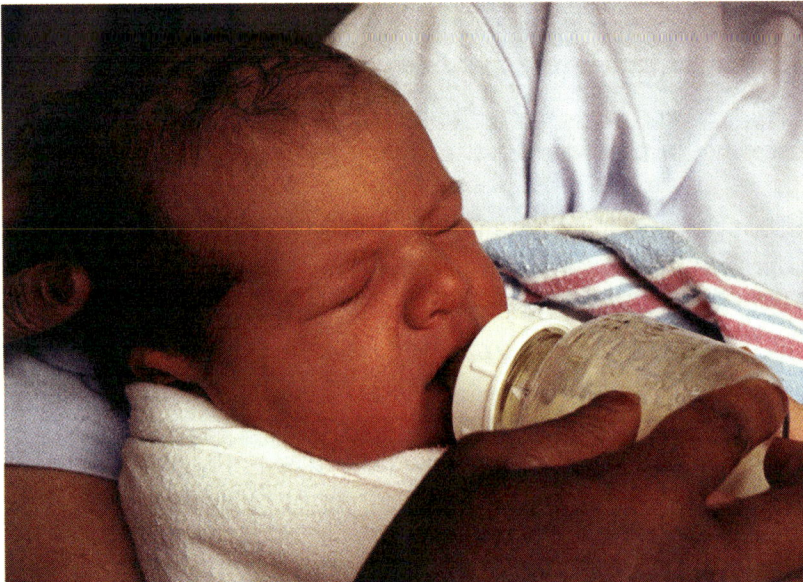

9-4 Holding your baby close during bottle-feedings can build a sense of comfort and trust.

Always refrigerate formula that has been prepared. Throw away any formula left in the bottle after a feeding. It can spoil easily and make the baby sick. Also discard any prepared formula that has been unrefrigerated for two hours or more. This formula may contain high levels of bacteria that grow quickly at room temperature.

Using the Bottle for Breast Milk

You can use the bottle to feed your baby breast milk if you like. For the first two to three weeks, however, don't introduce the bottle. Your baby does not suck in the same way at the breast as he does on the bottle. To nurse well, he needs to learn the jaw action that will get the milk from the breast. When you use both methods too soon, the baby may get confused. He may suck on the breast with the same motion he uses for the bottle. Not much milk will come out, which will frustrate both of you.

Using both methods too soon can also affect your milk supply. In the first few weeks, your body won't adjust well to changes in the demand for milk. Your system is regulated by how much breast milk the baby drinks. Each time he nurses, it tells your body to make more milk. If you use formula, your baby won't use all the milk your body makes. Your breasts may get hard and very sore. Your body will respond by making less milk. This may not be enough to meet his needs.

After a few weeks of breast-feeding, your body can better adapt your milk supply to your baby's needs. Then you should be able to introduce the bottle. The first time your baby tries a bottle, it might work best if someone else gives it to him. If you do it, he will be able to smell your milk and may want to nurse instead. It may take him a few tries to get used to the bottle, but soon he should be able to do both equally well.

Burping

Your baby needs to be burped during feedings. Babies swallow some air as they suck. This can cause discomfort and vomiting. Trapped air may make a baby feel full too soon. At first, burp your baby often to release this air. Breast-fed babies can be burped halfway through the feeding, or when you switch sides. For formula-fed infants, burp after every half- to one-ounce of formula. As they get older, most babies can be burped less frequently. If your baby spits up often, burping her more frequently may help.

To burp your baby, you can hold him in a sitting position on your lap. Gently rub or pat his upper back. (Use one hand on your baby's front to support his head and neck.) Another good position is to hold your baby against your shoulder. Place the baby's head and shoulders above your shoulder so he can breathe.

Sleep Needs

Newborns sleep most of the time. Your baby may sleep as many as 18 to 20 hours a day. As long as she wakes every three to four hours to eat, it's okay for her to sleep this much. She needs her rest because she is growing very quickly. If it has been more than four hours since your baby started her last feeding, you will need to wake her to eat. This is just a general guideline, however. Ask your baby's health care provider how often to feed her.

Gradually your baby will stay awake longer and sleep less. Your baby may stay awake at night and sleep during the day. Inside you, there was no night and day! You can slowly alter your baby's rhythm by playing with her after feedings or whenever she is awake during the day. This will keep her awake longer, and soon she will sleep more at night. See Figure 9-5.

During the day, it's a good idea not to keep the house unusually quiet. Your baby should get used to usual noises such as the TV, radio, vacuum cleaner, and voices. This way she will learn to sleep during usual household activities.

For a month or two, your baby will need to be fed more than once at night. It may be a few months before she sleeps all night. It will be hard for you to get enough sleep. To help, try resting during the day when your baby does. Lie down once or twice during the day, even if you don't sleep. You will be less tired and more patient with your baby if you get enough rest.

Schedules

It is not realistic to expect your newborn to be on a schedule. Your baby's needs change a little every day. You will only be frustrated if your plans depend on having him eat or sleep at a specific time. Plan to be flexible.

Allow your baby to guide you. He can let you know when he is hungry. When he is tired, he will sleep. In time, you will learn your baby's rhythm. Your baby's needs will become more predictable, too.

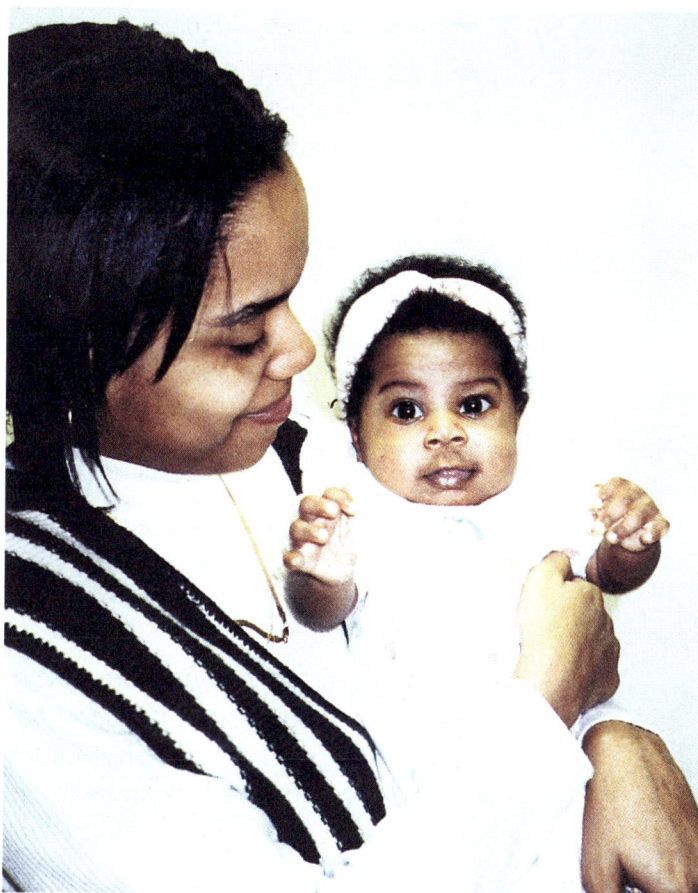

Bathing

Bathing your baby keeps her clean and healthy. You should use sponge baths to wash your newborn until the umbilical cord dries and falls off. (This should happen within a couple of weeks.) A bath every two to three days is fine. Your baby's hair needs to be washed only once or twice a week. Other times you can just wash her head with a warm, wet cloth.

9-5 Often, keeping your baby awake a little longer during the day will cause her to sleep longer at night.

Sponge Bath

To give a sponge bath, you will need the following equipment:

- a basin of water, if you are not near the sink
- baby soap and baby shampoo
- two towels—one to place under the baby and one for drying

- ☛ a soft wash cloth
- ☛ alcohol wipes or rubbing alcohol and cotton swabs to clean the stump of the umbilical cord (if recommended by your health care provider)
- ☛ sterile cotton balls
- ☛ clean clothes and diaper

Gather everything you need before undressing your baby. If the room is cool, use the towel to keep half of your baby warm while you bathe the other half. Wash your baby's face first with only warm water. Use clean water to moisten cotton balls and wipe her eyes.

Use soap and warm water to wash your baby's upper body (front and back). Be sure to clean all the skin folds, such as the neck and under the arms. Dry her upper body and put on a clean undershirt.

Next, wash the baby's lower body. Use care not to get the umbilical cord stump wet. It needs to dry out so it can fall off. Clean the baby's legs, feet, and diaper area with warm, soapy water. Use care to wash all the many skin folds of the legs and diaper area. Dry well to protect the baby's skin.

Put on a clean diaper. Fold down the front, top edge to leave the umbilical cord stump exposed to the air. If you cover the cord with the diaper, it won't dry out as fast. It will take longer to fall off and may get infected. After the diaper is on, wipe around the umbilical cord with an alcohol wipe or some alcohol on a cotton swab. (Some health care providers no longer recommend using alcohol on the umbilical cord—follow the advice of your baby's provider.) Let the cord dry well.

Tub Bath

Once the umbilical cord falls off, you may bathe your baby in a tub of warm water. If you want, you can use a baby bathtub. This is a small plastic tub you can place in or near a sink. See Figure 9-6. When buying a baby bathtub, look for a non-skid bottom, easy washability, and removable sponge pads. Be sure the tub has head and neck supports for your newborn. You'll also want a tub that is big enough to use for several months and is easy to carry and drain.

To give a tub bath, use just enough water for the baby to sit in. Test the water with your elbow to make sure it isn't too hot. (Your hands can stand hotter water than the baby can.) Cradle the baby in the curve of your left arm, so her head rests on your arm between your elbow and wrist. Now part of your arm will be under the baby's back. You can hold her left upper arm with your left hand. In this position, you have a firm grip on your baby. Your right hand is free to do the washing. If you are left-handed, you can reverse this hold.

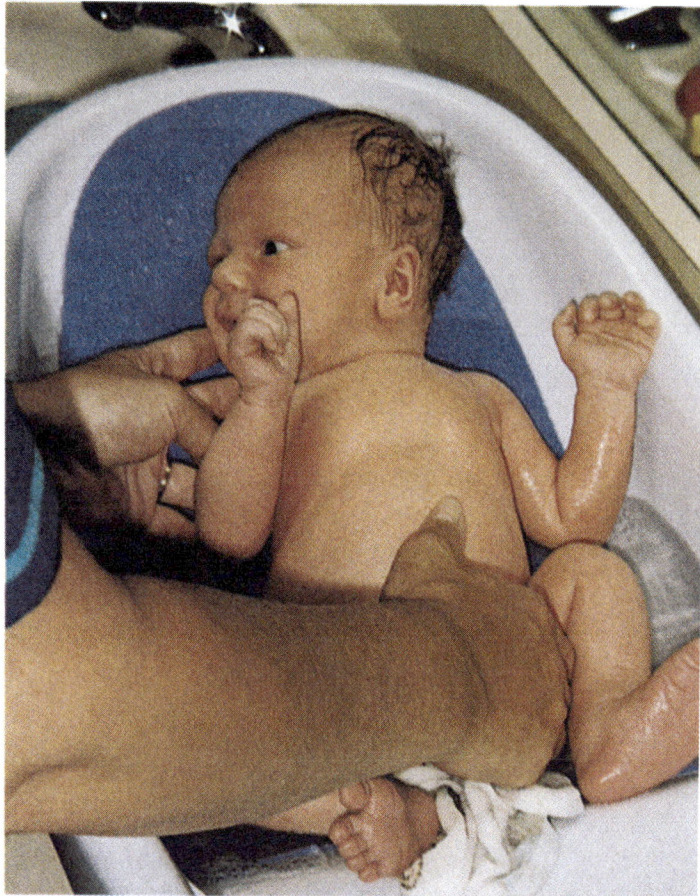

9-6 This plastic tub is good for bathing a baby who is a few weeks old. Newborns need sponge baths until the umbilical cord stump falls off.

After the bath, wrap your baby in a receiving blanket. This is a perfect time to play with your newborn, since she will be awake. If the bath made her fussy, a little attention should be very soothing. You may find a bath before bedtime helps your baby go to sleep.

Diapering

One of your most frequent activities as a new parent will be diapering your baby. Newborns need as many as 12 to 15 diaper changes daily. That's a lot of practice!

To keep your baby clean and dry, you can use either cloth or disposable diapers. Today, many parents prefer disposable diapers. They are convenient and easy to use. They don't need to be washed and don't require safety pins. Disposables are more expensive, however.

Cotton cloth diapers were once the standard. They are soft and absorbent. Cloth diapers can be washed and reused, which can make them more affordable. They don't create environmental waste. For these reasons, some parents prefer to use cloth diapers at least some of the time. Whichever you choose is fine. Your baby won't care as long as you keep his bottom clean and dry!

To change your baby's diaper, follow the steps given in Figure 9-7. Have everything you need nearby. When changing your baby, never leave him alone while you go to get something! You don't want to take even the smallest chance he could get hurt. Instead, take your baby with you.

It may be easiest to put everything you'll need in a diaper bag. This bag can come in handy at home and on the go. Look for a bag with multiple compartments (at least one waterproof), a zippered main compartment, a shoulder strap, and a detachable changing pad. An easy-to-clean or washable material is also preferred.

A baby's skin is very sensitive to moisture. Frequent diaper changes will prevent painful diaper rashes. Once a rash develops, it can be hard to get rid of it. Change your baby's diaper with each feeding and between feedings if it is wet or dirty. This will keep your baby clean, dry, and happy.

Baby's Bowel Movements

A newborn baby's first bowel movement (BM) is likely to be very soft and dark greenish-black in color. This is called meconium (muh-COH-nee-uhm). It is normal and may last several days. Gradually your baby's bowel movements will change. Formula-fed infants will have a harder, brown BM. Their BMs are less frequent than those of breast-fed babies. Many breast-fed babies have a BM every time

How to Diaper Your Baby

1. Gather everything you will need before you begin to change your baby. You will need the following:

   ❖ a clean diaper

   ❖ cotton balls and warm water or baby wipes

   ❖ a small towel or dry washcloth for drying

   ❖ a change of clothes for baby

   ❖ a protective cloth to put under baby

   Lotions and powders are not recommended. Lotions keep too much moisture on the baby's bottom. Babies can also be allergic to some of the ingredients in lotions. Powder is dangerous. Its tiny particles escape into the air and may be inhaled, causing lung problems.

2. Before you start, wash your hands or wipe them with a baby wipe.

3. Undo the tabs on the diaper and grasp your baby's feet in one hand, lifting them. With your other hand, pull the front of the diaper toward you. If your baby has had a bowel movement, use the clean edges of the diaper to wipe away as much stool as possible. (If the bowel movement is large and messy, it may be easier to carry the baby to a sink and wash the baby's bottom under warm running water.) Fold the clean surface of the diaper under the baby. Wash your baby's front with warm water or a baby wipe. Be sure to wipe from front to back. Make sure to clean the folds and creases of the skin. Lift baby's legs so you can clean the buttocks.

4. Pull the soiled diaper from under baby. If you use disposable diapers, fold the diaper with the contents inside and tape it closed with the tabs. This contains the odor and prevents spilling the contents.

5. Place a clean diaper under the baby and pat the baby dry with a towel. If you have a boy, cover his penis with a small cloth while you have the diaper off to prevent an unexpected spray of urine. It is a good idea to leave baby's bottom open to the air whenever possible to prevent diaper rash.

6. Pull the front of the diaper up and fasten closed with the tabs. Fold down the front so the umbilical cord stump is completely exposed.

7. Change any of the baby's clothes that were soiled.

8. Put the baby in a safe place. Wash your hands with warm, soapy water.

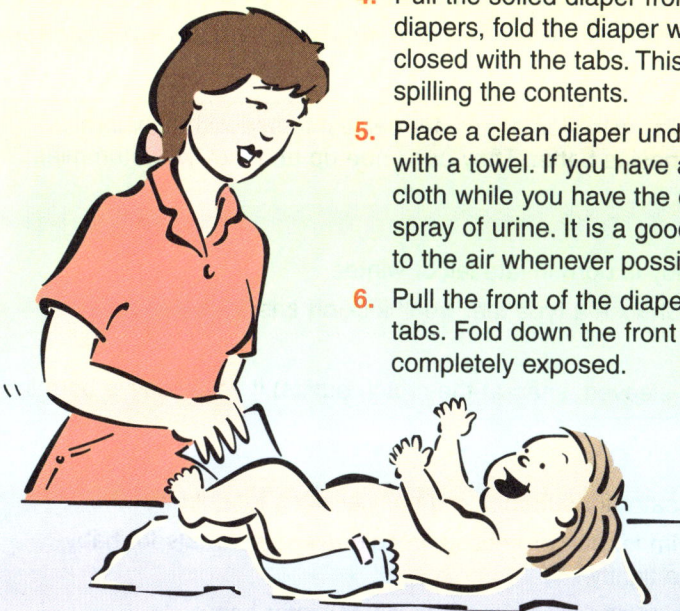

9-7 Changing diapers takes some practice, but soon it's easy for parents to do.

they nurse. These stools are likely to be a yellow color and very soft—sometimes almost liquid. Don't worry; this is not diarrhea. It happens because breast milk is more easily digested than formula.

How many BMs your baby has in a day is not important. The number varies from day to day and baby to baby. Over time, the number of daily stools will decrease. A day or two might even pass between BMs. This is normal. You only need to call the baby's health care provider if his BMs suddenly change in appearance or number. Also contact the provider if it has been a couple of days between BMs and the baby pulls at his legs or seems uncomfortable.

Dressing Your Baby

Dressing your baby can be fun. For the first few months, you will mainly need undershirts, nightgowns, and stretchies (one-piece outfits). See Figure 9-8 for a list of basic clothing for newborns.

How many you will need of each item depends on where you live. In a warm climate, you may never need heavy items such as snowsuits. How often you will wash clothes also makes a difference.

Basic Clothing for Newborns

* 3 to 7 undershirts. Front-open shirts with side snaps are easiest to use with newborns; after a few weeks you may like onesies better. They don't ride up and they keep tummies warm in cold weather.
* 3 to 8 nightgowns.
* 2 to 3 blanket sleepers if your baby is born in late fall or winter.
* 2 to 3 pairs of booties or socks. Choose a type that won't kick off easily.
* 3 to 6 stretchies with feet.
* 3 to 6 rompers (one-piece, short-sleeved, snap-at-the-crotch outfits) if your baby is born in late spring or summer.
* 2 to 3 washable bibs.
* 2 to 3 sweaters. 1 lightweight sweater for summer and heavier ones for cold weather.
* 1 to 3 hats. Lightweight with a brim for sun protection. In colder weather, hats for baby should cover the ears, but not too tightly.
* 1 bunting or snowsuit bag with mitts attached, for a late fall or winter baby.
* Diapers. 2 to 5 dozen cloth or several dozen disposables at one time.

9-8 Newborns need simple, comfortable clothing.

If you have easy access to a washing machine, you might wash every day. You wouldn't need as many clothes. However, if you wash only once a week, you'll need more of each item.

Babies grow quickly. To be on the safe side, buy clothes at least one size larger than your baby's age. For example, clothes size 3 to 6 months may fit some full-term newborns. Smaller newborns may need size 0 to 3 months clothes first. Premature infants may need clothes labeled <u>preemie</u> or <u>newborn</u>. Buying roomier clothes allows your baby to use them longer.

Cotton clothes are most comfortable for babies. They are also easy to wash. Keep in mind all-cotton clothes will shrink when you wash them. Always wash new baby's clothes in a mild detergent before putting them on your baby.

Buy clothes that are simple to put on and take off so you can easily change your baby's diaper. Clothes that slip over the head should have a wide opening at the neck. Avoid clothes with buttons. Clothes with snaps are much easier to manage.

Equipment for Baby

Many stores and magazines sell baby products. They offer a huge selection of baby clothes, equipment, and supplies. These items can be very attractive, but the cost can add up quickly. You might imagine your baby in a brand new crib. If you can afford it, that's great! If not, a safe secondhand crib works just as well. Besides a crib, there are some other basic items you'll need. Some of them you may be able to borrow from family and friends. Others you will need to buy.

This section describes the baby equipment you will need. Each item has its own unique safety features. A few general points apply, however. The following are important to look for when buying baby equipment:

- lead-free paint (lead can poison the baby)
- sturdy, non-tip construction
- smooth edges and rounded corners
- restraint straps (where appropriate)

Do a safety check on all baby items before you purchase them. Avoid sharp points or small parts that might break loose. Check for exposed hinges or springs. Watch for attached strings, cords, or ribbons that could strangle the baby. It's your job to keep your newborn safe and healthy.

Baby Furnishings

You will have to decide where baby will sleep. In some families, a baby will have a separate room. Many teen moms live at home with their families, though. They share their bedrooms with their babies. If you and your baby will share a room, you may need to rearrange to make space for the baby's things. Your newborn doesn't need much room. She will need a bed and space to store her clothes, toys, and other equipment.

The most important furnishing your baby will need is a place to sleep. Most parents choose to use a crib. You could also use a bassinet, which is a small basketlike bed. This would take up less room, but baby would outgrow it within a few months. Some mothers have their newborns sleep in bed with them. For safety reasons, this is not recommended. You might accidentally roll onto the baby, smother her, or cause her to fall out of bed. This is too dangerous a risk.

When choosing a crib, keep safety points in mind. You might consider a used crib that you could borrow or buy at a garage sale or used furniture store. Do not use any crib that was made before 1988. (If in doubt, choose another crib.) Cribs this old do not meet current safety standards. Look for a label on your crib stating that Consumer Product Safety Commission (CPSC) standards have been met. Additional safety features to look for in a crib are listed in Figure 9-9.

What you place inside the crib is just as important. First, you will need a set of bumper pads to keep baby from hitting herself on the crib rails. The bumper pads should fit snugly around the entire inside of the crib. They should have at least six ties or sets of snaps for fastening them to the crib rails. A list of other bedding

Choosing a Crib

When selecting a crib for your baby, check for the following:

❖ no splinters or cracks in the crib frame

❖ space between rails measures no more than 2⅜ inches so baby can't get her arm, leg, or head stuck (the space is too wide if a soft drink can fits between the slats)

❖ crib mattress fits snugly in the crib—space between crib and mattress measures no more than two adult finger-widths (so baby doesn't get stuck)

❖ mattress height can be lowered as baby grows and top of rail is 26 inches from top of mattress at the highest level (keeps baby from crawling or falling out)

❖ plastic teething rails are tightly secured and unbroken

9-9 When shopping for a crib, there are several key points to keep in mind.

you will need is given in Figure 9-10. Be sure not to put any pillows or stuffed animals in bed with the baby for the first year. These can suffocate her.

You will also need a place to store your baby's belongings. Clothes, toys, and equipment can take up more space than you might think. You may be able to share a chest of drawers with baby, or she might need one of her own. This will depend on the space and money available, as well as how many items the baby has. Open, stackable crates or shelves can also be useful. If you organize your space well, you can probably make plenty of room for your new baby.

Basic Bedding Items

❖ 3 to 6 receiving blankets
❖ 3 to 4 fitted crib sheets
❖ 2 quilted mattress pads (optional)
❖ 2 to 6 waterproof pads, in two sizes for protecting cribs, stroller, laps, and furniture
❖ 1 to 2 washable crib blankets
❖ 1 to 2 smaller blankets for stroller

9-10 Your baby needs a few basic bedding items. If it's very cold where you live, heavier blankets may be needed.

Outing Equipment

Babies do not stay indoors all the time. You'll have places to go and things to do. Often your baby will go with you. Therefore, you'll need some type of outing equipment for him. Exactly what you will need depends upon your lifestyle. Some of the items you might need are a car seat, stroller or carriage, and an infant carrier.

Car Safety Seat

When your baby rides in a car, he must be securely fastened in an approved car safety seat. This is the law in every state. A neck support should be used with the car seat for the first few months. You can use a rolled towel or buy a special cloth neck support. Some car seats come with a built-in neck support you can remove when the baby is older. See Figure 9-11.

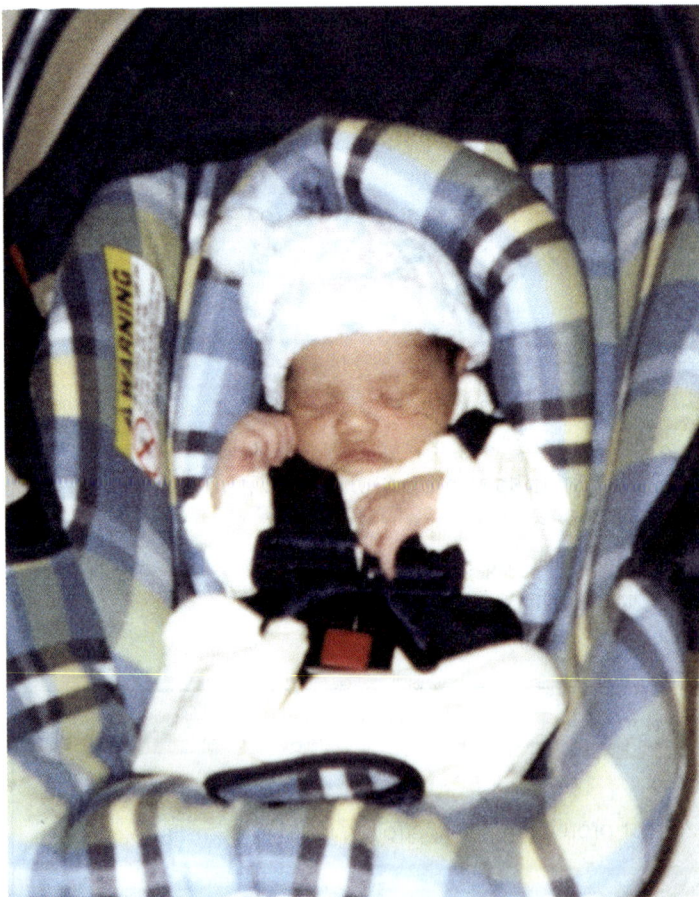

9-11 The built-in neck support in this car seat provides the added protection this very young baby needs. If your car seat doesn't have this, you can use a rolled towel or infant neck support pillow instead.

You may use either an infant seat or convertible seat. An infant seat faces backward and uses a reclining position. It is for babies weighing less than 20 to 22 pounds. A convertible seat can be used for babies up to 40 pounds. It can recline and face backward for infant use. When your baby is older, this seat can be switched to an upright, front-facing position.

When shopping for a car safety seat, read the label for age recommendations.

Look for the Juvenile Products Manufacturing Association (JPMA) certification seal of approval. Choose a model that is easy to install and remove. Look for a one-latch harness. This type of restraint makes it easier to fasten and release your baby. Consider your baby's comfort. A washable padding or easy-to-clean surface is also good.

Stroller

Suppose you want to take your baby on outings where you will be walking. You will probably need a stroller. What type should you get? This depends upon how often you'll use it and where you will go. If you live in a city and use public transportation, you may want a lightweight, foldable stroller. In a rural or suburban area, you might want a bigger, sturdier model for walks through the neighborhood. Look for a stroller that will meet your specific needs.

Check the label for the age recommendations and the JPMA certification seal. This means the product has been tested and approved. Look for a reclining seat. This makes the stroller useful for a very young infant and for naps when your baby is older. Secure and easy-to-fasten restraining straps are important. So are large wheels that allow a stroller to turn more easily.

For safety, choose a stroller with a sun shield; broad, non-tip base; good brakes; and hinges that won't catch curious fingers. A comfortable handle height and package rack can make a stroller easier for parents to use. You may want a stroller that is easy to fold and carry.

Don't be afraid to test a stroller before you buy it. This is the best way to know if you will like it. Practice putting your baby in and taking him out. Push the stroller around the store. Testing strollers will help you find the right one for you.

Infant Carriers

You may also want to have an infant carrier for your baby. There are two main types of carriers. One is somewhat like an infant car seat. It is a plastic seat with restraint straps and a handle for easy carrying. This infant carrier also makes a good indoor or outdoor seat. Look for wide, sturdy, stable base and a non-skid or suction bottom. Infant carrier seats should <u>not</u> be used as car seats. They do not meet the safety standards to be used in this way.

Another type of infant carrier is made of cloth. You can wear this carrier to keep baby close to your body. This makes it convenient to carry your baby at home or away because your hands are free. Look for a front carrier model. (A baby is too young for a back carrier until he can sit independently.) Choose one that is easy to fasten and detach without help. Check for adjustable, padded straps that are comfortable. Find one that offers head and neck support for baby and a wide bottom to support baby's bottom and thighs.

These are the items you will likely need for your newborn. As your baby gets older, your equipment needs will change.

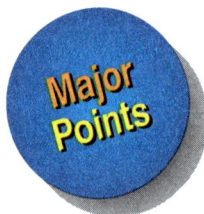

Major Points

☞ Medical care is an important part of caring for your newborn. You and your baby's health care provider can work together to keep your newborn healthy. Taking your baby for scheduled checkups and immunizations is important.

☞ Feeding your new baby is one of your most important jobs. Whether you decide to breast-feed or bottle-feed, learn about your method. Know how to feed your baby correctly—this will keep your baby healthy and safe.

☞ Your newborn may sleep most of the day. As long as he or she wakes for feedings, this is okay. Your baby should eat at least every four hours.

☞ It is not realistic to expect your newborn to be on a schedule. Your baby's needs will change a little every day. Plan to be flexible.

☞ Until your baby's umbilical cord falls off, give your baby sponge baths. In a few weeks, the baby will be ready for tub baths. You can buy a special baby bathtub if you wish.

☛   Babies have sensitive skin. Frequent diaper changes will help them avoid diaper rash. Diapering is a skill you will quickly develop. Your newborn may need as many as 12 to 15 changes daily!

☛   Dressing your baby can be fun. Choose clothes carefully to meet your baby's needs. Clothes with snaps down the front and inside the legs are easier to use.

☛   Babies need some furnishings, such as a crib. They also need equipment for outings. Examine any baby supplies carefully for sturdiness and safety. Make sure these items are approved. In every state, it is a law babies must be fastened in an approved car safety seat for each car ride.

Glossary

A

abstinence. Choosing to postpone sex until a time in a person's life when he or she is ready to enter this type of relationship. (8)

active labor. The second phase of stage one of labor; occurs between early labor and transition; cervix dilates to 7 or 8 cm. (7)

afterbirth. The name for the placenta and other pregnancy-related tissues that are expelled from the uterus in the third stage of labor. (7)

afterbirth pains. Contractions of the uterus that occur for a few days after childbirth. (8)

amniocentesis. Prenatal test in which a small amount of amniotic fluid is taken and tested to find any physical problems with an unborn baby. (4)

amniotic fluid. Fluid in the amniotic sac that protects the baby, regulates the baby's temperature, and gives the baby freedom to move. (3)

amniotic sac. Thin membrane that surrounds an unborn baby and holds amniotic fluid; also called the bag of waters. (3)

analgesia. Type of pain medication that reduces pain and discomfort throughout the entire body. (7)

anemia. Condition caused by lack of iron in the blood; it is common during pregnancy, but can be dangerous to the woman and her unborn baby. (4)

anesthesia. Type of pain medication that takes pain away completely in a given area. (7)

anonymous testing. Type of medical test in which no one knows the identity of the person taking the test; commonly used when testing for pregnancy or STIs. (2)

antibodies. Substances that help the body fight disease. (6)

Apgar score. Score given on the Apgar test, which tests a newborn's condition within a few minutes after birth. (8)

areola. Darker area around the nipple. (3)

B

bacterial vaginosis. A condition linked to sexual intercourse, but not contracted from a partner. It has been associated with premature birth and infection inside the uterus and amniotic sac. (4)

baby blues. Common feelings mothers have after childbirth that may include sadness, crying, and frustration. These feelings last a short time and go away on their own. (8)

babysitting. Type of child care that lasts a few hours in a single day. (6)

bag of waters. Another name for the <u>amniotic sac</u>. (3)

bimanual. Physical exam of the female reproductive organs in which the health care provider inserts two fingers into a woman's vagina and rests the other hand on top of her abdomen. (4)

birth certificate. Legal document that proves a baby was born and provides information about the birth. (8)

bloody show. Another name for the show; a pink-tinged discharge that happens close to labor when the mucus plug is released from the cervix. (7)

bonding. Unique strong attachment that develops between parents and their baby. (8)

Braxton-Hicks contractions. Another name for false labor contractions that may occur on and off toward the end of pregnancy. (7)

breech position. Position in which the baby is feet-first or sitting down against the cervix; this position sometimes requires a cesarean delivery. (7)

C

certified nurse-midwife. Nurse who is trained to give prenatal care and can deliver babies. (4)

cervix. Narrow, muscular opening at the bottom of the uterus. (1)

cesarean delivery. Operation in which the baby is born through a cut in the mother's uterus and abdomen; done when a vaginal birth is dangerous or impossible. (7)

cesarean section. Another name for <u>cesarean delivery</u>. (7)

C-section. Another name for <u>cesarean delivery</u>. (7)

childbirth. A process through which a baby is born. (7)

chromosomes. Parts of cells that carry the traits parents pass on to their children. (3)

circumcision. Surgical procedure in which part of the loose foreskin of the male penis is removed. (8)

clitoris. Small, sensitive organ that provides sexual arousal in the female and is part of the vulva. (1)

colostrum. Thick yellow fluid produced by the breasts for the first few days after birth. This fluid is rich in nutrients and antibodies. (9)

conception. The union of an egg and sperm cell; also called <u>fertilization</u>. (1)

conditioning. A type of exercise that makes muscles stronger and better able to do continued work. (5)

confidential testing. Type of medical test in which the identity of the person taking the test is known. (2)

constipation. Condition in which a person is unable to have a bowel movement or has hard stools. (3)

contraction. The name for a tightening and relaxing of the muscles of the uterus; can signal either false or true labor. (7)

crowning. The moment when the baby's head can be seen at the opening of the birth canal. (7)

D

dehydration. Condition in which the body's fluid level is too low. (2)

delivery. The actual movement of baby and the placenta from the uterus out of the mother's body. (7)

diabetes. An illness in which a person's body cannot use sugar in the right way. (4)

dilatation. The process through which the cervix opens during labor. (7)

doctor. A person who has earned a medical degree. (4)

doula. A person trained to be a labor supporter. (6)

due date. The estimated date your baby will be born. (4)

E

ectopic pregnancy. Pregnancy in which the fertilized egg attaches somewhere other than the uterus and begins to grow. (2)

effacement. Term that describes the shortening and thinning of the cervix. (7)

egg. Female reproductive cell. Its job is to unite with a sperm cell to create a baby. (1)

ejaculation. A process of muscle contractions that push semen out of the body. (1)

ejaculatory duct. Small duct that connects the seminal vesicles to the urethra. Sperm enter here just before ejaculation. (1)

embryo. Name for unborn baby from implantation to eight weeks after conception. (3)

endometrium. Lining of the uterus on which blood and tissues build to nourish a fertilized egg. In pregnancy, the baby will attach here. (1)

engage. To settle into position against the mother's pelvic bone in preparation for birth; done by the fetus during the ninth month of pregnancy. (3)

engorgement. Painful condition in which a woman's breasts become overfull with milk, swell, harden, and become sore. (8)

enriched. Type of food product in which nutrients have been added to it. (5)

epididymis. Organ in which the sperm mature. (1)

epidural. Type of regional anesthesia that is injected into the spinal cord during labor; it numbs the mother from the waist down. (7)

episiotomy. Small cut made at the opening of the birth canal to widen it so the baby has enough room to be delivered. (7)

erection. Process by which a man's penis becomes harder, wider, and longer. Happens when spongy tissue inside the penis fills with blood. (1)

esophagus. Long thin tube that carries food from the mouth to the stomach. (3)

express. To pump out milk from the breast. (6)

F

failure to progress. Term used to describe labor that is not going as it should; can be cause to do a C-section. (7)

fallopian tubes. Two tubes in which eggs travel from the ovaries to the uterus. (1)

false labor. Name for contractions that occur toward the end of pregnancy that do not signal that labor has started; also called Braxton-Hicks contractions. (7)

family practice doctor. Type of doctor who treats all kinds of patients but has enough education and training to give prenatal care and deliver babies. (4)

fertilization. The union of a sperm and egg cell; also called conception. (1)

fetal alcohol syndrome (FAS). Condition that occurs in babies of mothers who drink alcohol heavily during pregnancy; includes various lasting physical and mental disabilities. (4)

fetal distress. Term used to describe a fetus during labor who has an abnormally slow heartbeat and isn't getting enough oxygen; can be cause to do a C-section. (7)

fetus. Name for an unborn baby from the ninth week of pregnancy until birth. (3)

foreskin. Looser skin that covers the penis and may be removed by circumcision. (1)

full-term. Describing a baby whose prenatal development is complete; a pregnancy that lasts more than 37 weeks. (3)

fundal height. The distance from the top of the uterus to the bottom; measurement taken at prenatal visits to see if the baby has grown. (4)

G

general anesthesia. Type of medication that numbs the entire body and puts a person to sleep; used only in emergency cesarean deliveries. (7)

gestational diabetes. Type of diabetes that can develop during pregnancy and go away after delivery. (4)

glans. Smooth, round tip of the penis. (1)

H

health care provider. A person or agency qualified to provide medical care. This might be a family doctor, certified nurse-midwife, health department, or clinic. (2)

heartburn. A burning sensation in the chest caused by stomach acid flowing backward into the esophagus. (3)

hemorrhoids. Swollen veins in the rectum caused by straining to have a bowel movement or straining to push during delivery. (3)

I

immunization. Medicine given, usually in an injection (shot), to prevent serious diseases from developing. (9)

implantation. Attachment of a hollow ball of cells to the endometrium in the uterus. (1)

incubator. Special bed that keeps germs and cold from harming a baby in an intensive care unit. Often used for premature or low-birthweight babies. (8)

iron-fortified. Type of infant formula that has had iron added to it. This is the kind of formula newborns need. (6)

K

Kegel exercise. Conditioning exercise done by contracting and relaxing the pelvic floor muscles. (5)

L

labia majora. Two hairy outer liplike flaps of skin that protect the vaginal opening. These are parts of the vulva. (1)

labia minora. Two hairless inner liplike flaps of skin that protect the vaginal opening. These are parts of the vulva. (1)

labor. The work the uterus and cervix do to prepare for delivering a baby. (7)

labor helper. Person who will be with you during childbirth classes, labor, and delivery. (6)

lactation specialist. Professional who teaches women about breast-feeding. People in this career usually work in hospitals. (6)

La Leche League. An organization that supports breast-feeding. This group helps new mothers, as well as providing breast-feeding classes. (6)

lanugo. Fine, soft hair that grows on the fetus during the fifth month of pregnancy. (3)

latch-on. The hold a baby's mouth has on the mother's breast. Should include the nipple and much of the areola. (9)

lightening. A sensation caused when the baby engages its head against the pelvic bone and drops lower in the mother's abdomen when birth is near. (7)

local anesthesia. Type of medicine that numbs only a very small area; may be used to numb the birth canal for an episiotomy or to stitch the cut after one. (7)

lochia. Discharge from the vagina that occurs after childbirth. (8)

low birthweight. Describes a baby who weighs less than 5 ½ pounds at birth. (4)

M

mask of pregnancy. Condition in which the facial skin darkens during pregnancy and lightens slowly after delivery. (3)

mastitis. An infection of a milk duct in the breast that can be identified by a sore, red spot on the breast or fever. (8)

maternal serum alpha-fetoprotein test (MSAFP). Blood test of the mother to screen for Down syndrome and problems with the baby's brain and spinal cord. (4)

mature milk. Thin bluish-white fluid the breasts produce once breast-feeding is well established. (9)

meconium. Baby's first bowel movement; is soft with a greenish-black color. (9)

Medicaid. Government program that provides free medical care to those who cannot afford it and meet the qualifications. (2)

menstrual cycle. A series of monthly body changes in females that prepares the body for possible pregnancy. (1)

menstrual period. Another name for menstruation. (1)

menstruation. Shedding of unneeded blood and tissues that have built up on the endometrium; also called the menstrual period or period. (1)

miscarriage. The body's way to end a pregnancy before its fifth month. (2)

morning sickness. Common name for nausea and vomiting in pregnancy; happens most often in the morning, but can happen any time of day or night. (3)

mucus plug. Mucus that fills the cervix to protect the baby during pregnancy and comes out during labor. (7)

MyPyramid. A personalized system that helps you plan a nutritious diet. (5)

N

nurse practitioner. A nurse who has special training in women's health; abbreviated NP. An NP can give prenatal care but cannot deliver babies. (4)

nursing. Another name for breast-feeding. (6)

nutrient. A chemical substance found in food that helps build and maintain the body. (5)

O

obstetrician. A doctor who specializes in prenatal care and childbirth. (4)

ovaries. Two small, almond-shaped organs that produce and store eggs in the female. (1)

over-the-counter (OTC) drugs. Medications that can be bought without a prescription from a doctor; can be dangerous to an unborn baby if the mother takes them. (4)

ovulation. The process that includes an ovary releasing a mature egg. (1)

P

Pap test. Test that involves collecting cervical cells and testing them for cancer. (4)

passive smoking. Inhaling smoke from someone's lit cigarette; can be dangerous to an unborn baby. (4)

pediatrician. A doctor who specializes in caring for babies and children. (6)

pelvic floor muscles. A group of muscles that support a woman's bladder, uterus, and bowel. These muscles should be conditioned during pregnancy. (5)

pelvic inflammatory disease (PID). Disease in which the female reproductive organs become infected and inflamed; a common cause of ectopic pregnancy. (2)

pelvic tilt exercise. Conditioning exercise that is done to relieve backache. (5)

penis. Organ that enters a woman's vagina during sex. Semen and urine leave the body from the urethra inside the penis. (1)

PET. An abbreviation for preeclampsia/toxemia. (4)

placenta. Organ that acts as an exchange site between a pregnant woman and her baby. (3)

placenta previa. A condition in which the placenta covers the cervix, blocking the baby from entering the birth canal; may result in a cesarean delivery. (7)

postpartum depression. Condition of serious depression experienced after childbirth. This condition is rare and needs medical attention. (8)

postpartum period. Period of six weeks immediately following childbirth during which the mother recovers. (8)

preeclampsia. High-risk pregnancy condition that starts with a sudden rise in the mother's blood pressure; also called toxemia or PET. (4)

premature labor. Labor that begins before week 37 of pregnancy. (4)

prenatal care. Medical care given during pregnancy. (4)

prenatal development. A baby's growth and development before birth. (3)

prepared childbirth. Childbirth in which no medication is used; instead the woman relies on breathing and relaxation exercises she learned in a childbirth class. (7)

prostate gland. Plum-sized gland that adds fluid to semen. (1)

puberty. The process through which a person's reproductive organs mature and become able to create new life. This happens in adolescence. (1)

pubic mound. A fatty pad of tissue that covers and protects the pubic bone in women. It is part of the vulva. (1)

R

regional anesthesia. Type of anesthesia which numbs only one region of the body, but doesn't make the person fall asleep. (7)

reproductive system. The body system containing the parts and pathways that allow a person to bear children. (1)

Rh factor. A substance in the blood that people either have (Rh+) or do not have (Rh-). If a pregnant woman is Rh- and her baby is Rh+, it can cause problems. (4)

role model. A person whose actions are copied by others. (6)

S

scrotum. Sac of loose skin that hangs down just behind the penis and holds the testes. (1)

secondhand smoke. Smoke a person inhales from another person's cigarette; can be dangerous to a baby during pregnancy and after birth. (4)

semen. Mixture that contains sperm and fluids from the prostate gland and seminal vesicles. (1)

seminal vesicles. Two small glands that add fluid to sperm to make semen. (1)

sexually transmitted diseases (STDs). A name that is sometimes used to describe sexually transmitted infections. (4)

sexually transmitted infections (STIs). Infections that are spread from one person to another during sexual activity. (4)

shaft. Longest part of the penis. (1)

show. A pink-tinged discharge that happens close to labor when the mucus plug is released from the cervix. (7)

sonogram. Picture of an unborn baby; created by sound waves in an ultrasound test. (4)

Special Supplemental Nutrition Program for Women, Infants, and Children (WIC). A federally-funded government program that offers food vouchers and counseling on nutrition and breast-feeding; available to pregnant or breast-feeding women, as well as their infants and children. (5)

speculum. A medical instrument that is inserted into the vagina to hold it open; used to allow the health care provider to examine the vagina and cervix. (4)

sperm. Male reproductive cell. Its function is to unite with an egg cell to make a baby. (1)

stretch marks. Dark, reddish marks that appear on the skin of the abdomen, buttocks, and breasts; caused by tearing of the tissue under the skin as the skin stretches. (3)

swaddling. Gently wrapping a thin blanket snugly around your baby for comfort. (8)

T

testes. Two small, walnut-shaped organs located inside the scrotum that produce sperm and testosterone. (1)

testosterone. Hormone that controls puberty in men and signals young men's bodies to begin making sperm. (1)

toxemia. Another name for preeclampsia. (4)

transition. Last phase of stage one of labor; occurs between active labor and stage two of labor; hardest part of labor. (7)

transitional milk. Type of milk that is present from a few days after labor until two to three weeks after labor. (9)

trimesters. Three parts of pregnancy, each lasting about 3 months or 13 weeks. (3)

tubal pregnancy. Type of ectopic pregnancy that implants in the fallopian tubes. This is a medical emergency. (2)

U

ultrasound test. Test that uses sound waves to make a video image of an unborn baby; can detect physical disabilities, tell the baby's gender, and estimate the due date. (4)

umbilical cord. Thick, flexible cord that contains three blood vessels. It connects the placenta and the baby. (3)

urethra. In males, the tube inside the penis that carries urine and semen out of the body. In females, the tube that carries urine out of the body. (1)

urinary opening. Small opening in the woman's body where urine leaves the body. It is not part of the vulva. (1)

urinary tract infection (UTI). An infection of the bladder, urethra, or other part of the urinary system. (2)

uterus. Muscular, pear-shaped organ where a baby grows until birth; also called the womb. (1)

V

vagina. Muscular tunnel that leads from the cervix to the outside of the body; also called the birth canal. (1)

vaginal birth. Birth in which the mother pushes the baby out of her uterus and out of her birth canal. (7)

varicose veins. Condition of swollen and enlarged blood vessels in the legs. (3)

vas deferens. Two long, thin tubes that store sperm until they are released from the body in an ejaculation. (1)

vernix. White, waxy coating that covers a baby's skin in the fifth month of pregnancy. (3)

vulva. The group of a woman's external reproductive organs; includes the pubic mound, the labia minora and majora, and the clitoris. (1)

W

womb. Another name for the uterus. (1)

WIC. A federally-funded government program that offers nutrition and breast-feeding counseling. Available to pregnant or breast-feeding women, or their infants and children. (5)

Z

zygote. Single cell created by the union of sperm and egg. It contains all the information it needs to grow into a baby. (1)

Index